GIANT CELL ARTERITIS DIET COOKBOOK

Tasty Treats for Arteritis Management

Dr. Melissa R. Steven

INTRODUCTION

Welcome to the Giant Cell Arteritis Diet Cookbook, a comprehensive guide designed to support individuals managing Giant Cell Arteritis (GCA) through the power of nutrition. This cookbook is crafted with the understanding that dietary choices can play a significant role in managing the symptoms and promoting overall health for those living with GCA.

Giant Cell Arteritis is an inflammatory condition affecting the arteries, particularly those in the head and neck, which can lead to severe complications if not managed effectively. While medical treatments are crucial, adopting a balanced and nutritious diet tailored to GCA can complement traditional therapies and improve quality of life.

In this cookbook, you will find a wealth of recipes meticulously curated to incorporate anti-inflammatory ingredients and support optimal nutrition. From nourishing breakfasts to satisfying main dishes, wholesome snacks, and refreshing beverages, each recipe is crafted with both taste and health benefits in mind.

Beyond recipes, this book offers essential guidance on meal planning, grocery shopping tips, batch cooking strategies, and special dietary considerations such as gluten-free, dairy-free, and vegetarian options. You will also discover insights into the role of specific nutrients and supplements in GCA management, empowering you to make informed choices about your diet.

Whether you are newly diagnosed or seeking new ways to enhance your well-being, this cookbook aims to inspire and support you on your journey towards better health. By embracing delicious, nutrient-dense meals and adopting mindful eating practices, you can take proactive steps in managing GCA and living a vibrant, fulfilling life.

Let this cookbook be your companion in nourishing both body and spirit as you navigate the path to wellness with Giant Cell Arteritis.

Here's to good health and flavorful eating!

TABLE OF CONTENTS

1.1 What is Giant Cell Arteritis?

Giant Cell Arteritis (GCA), also known as temporal arteritis or cranial arteritis, is a type of vasculitis that involves inflammation of the blood vessels, primarily the large and medium-sized arteries in the head and neck. This condition is characterized by the presence of abnormally large cells, known as giant cells, within the walls of the affected arteries. GCA predominantly affects individuals over the age of 50 and is more common in women and people of Northern European descent.

The inflammation caused by GCA can lead to narrowing or blockage of the arteries, reducing blood flow and potentially causing serious complications, such as vision loss or stroke. The exact cause of GCA is not fully understood, but it is believed to involve a combination of genetic and environmental factors that trigger an abnormal immune response. Diagnosis typically involves clinical evaluation, blood tests to check for inflammation, imaging studies, and a biopsy of the temporal artery to confirm the presence of giant cells and other inflammatory changes.

1.2 The Role of Diet in Managing Giant Cell Arteritis

Diet plays a significant role in managing Giant Cell Arteritis (GCA) by helping to reduce inflammation, manage symptoms, and support overall health. Incorporating anti-inflammatory foods such as fruits, vegetables, whole grains, healthy fats, lean proteins, nuts, and seeds can help alleviate inflammation. On the other hand, avoiding processed foods, refined carbohydrates, sugary beverages, red and processed meats, and trans fats is crucial to prevent exacerbating inflammation. Nutritional supplements like omega-3 fatty acids, vitamin D, and calcium can also support the dietary management of GCA. Staying well-hydrated and maintaining a healthy weight are additional factors that contribute to effective dietary management of the condition. Through mindful dietary choices, individuals with GCA can significantly enhance their overall well-being and complement their medical treatment.

1.3 How to Use This Cookbook

This cookbook is designed to be your comprehensive guide to managing Giant Cell Arteritis (GCA) through nutrition. This is the way to take full advantage of it:

Understanding GCA and Nutrition

Begin by reading the sections on understanding GCA and the importance of nutrition in managing the condition. These chapters provide essential information on how diet impacts inflammation and overall health.

Exploring Nutrition Basics

Familiarize yourself with the basics of an anti-inflammatory diet. Learn about the foods that help reduce inflammation and those that should be avoided. This foundation will help you make informed choices as you plan your meals.

Meal Planning and Preparation

Use the meal planning and preparation chapters to organize your meals efficiently. You'll find tips on meal planning, grocery shopping, and batch cooking. These strategies are designed to save time and ensure you always have healthy, anti-inflammatory meals ready to go.

Recipes for Every Meal

Explore the recipe sections for breakfast, lunch, dinner, snacks, appetizers, desserts, and beverages. Each recipe is crafted to be delicious, nutritious, and supportive of your health goals. The recipes are categorized to help you easily find options for different meals and occasions.

Special Diets and Modifications

If you have specific dietary needs, such as gluten-free, dairy-free, vegetarian, or vegan, refer to the special diets and modifications section. Here, you'll find tailored recipes and tips to accommodate your dietary preferences while still adhering to an anti-inflammatory diet.

Sample Meal Plans

Get started with our sample meal plans, whether you're a beginner or looking for advanced options. These plans provide structured guidance to help you integrate the principles of an anti-inflammatory diet into your daily routine.

Tips for Dining Out

Learn how to make healthy choices when eating out with the tips for dining out section. This chapter offers advice on selecting anti-inflammatory options at restaurants and packing meals for travel.

Mindful Eating and Lifestyle Tips

Enhance your overall well-being by incorporating mindful eating practices, stress management techniques, and physical activity. The mindful eating and lifestyle tips section provides practical advice to support a holistic approach to managing GCA.

Using the Cookbook as a Daily Resource

Keep this cookbook handy as a daily resource. Refer to it when planning meals, shopping for groceries, or seeking inspiration for new recipes. Use it as a tool to stay motivated and committed to a diet that supports your health and helps manage GCA.

By following the guidance and recipes in this cookbook, you can take an active role in managing Giant Cell Arteritis through nutrition. Enjoy the journey to better health and delicious, anti-inflammatory meals!

Understanding Giant Cell Arteritis

2.1 Symptoms and Diagnosis

Giant Cell Arteritis (GCA) can present with a wide range of symptoms, often making it challenging to diagnose. The most **common symptoms include:**

1. Headache: A persistent, severe headache, often located at the temples or the back of the head. This is the most characteristic symptom of GCA.
Scalp Tenderness: Increased sensitivity or pain when touching or brushing the scalp.
2. Jaw Claudication: Pain and fatigue in the jaw muscles while chewing or talking. This occurs due to reduced blood flow to the muscles of the jaw.
3. Visual Disturbances: Blurred vision, double vision, or sudden, temporary, or permanent vision loss. These symptoms result from inflammation of the arteries that supply the eyes.
4. Systemic Symptoms: Fever, fatigue, unintentional weight loss, night sweats, and muscle aches. These systemic symptoms reflect the body's inflammatory response.
5. Polymyalgia Rheumatica: Many patients with GCA also have polymyalgia rheumatica, which causes pain and stiffness in the shoulders, hips, and neck.

Less common symptoms include:

- Peripheral Artery Symptoms: Pain or weakness in the limbs due to reduced blood flow.
- Neurological Symptoms: Stroke or transient ischemic attacks (TIAs) due to inflammation of the arteries supplying the brain.

Diagnosis

Diagnosing GCA involves a combination of clinical evaluation, laboratory tests, and imaging studies. Early and accurate diagnosis is critical to prevent serious complications, such as vision loss and stroke.

1. Medical History and Physical Examination: A detailed medical history and physical examination are the first steps. The doctor will look for characteristic symptoms and signs, such as tenderness of the temporal arteries.

2. Blood Tests: Elevated levels of inflammatory markers, such as erythrocyte sedimentation rate (ESR) and C-reactive protein (CRP), are common in GCA. These tests demonstrate the presence of aggravation in the body.

3. Imaging Studies: Ultrasound of the temporal arteries can show signs of inflammation, such as a "halo sign," which is a dark area around the artery indicating swelling. Magnetic resonance imaging (MRI) or positron emission tomography (PET) scans can also be used to detect inflammation in larger arteries.

4. Temporal Artery Biopsy: This is the gold standard for diagnosing GCA. A small sample of the temporal artery is surgically removed and examined under a microscope. The presence of giant cells and other inflammatory changes confirms the diagnosis. However, a negative biopsy does not completely rule out GCA, as the inflammation can be patchy.

5. Additional Tests: In some cases, other tests may be performed to assess the extent of the disease and rule out other conditions. These might include angiography to visualize the arteries or echocardiography to check for involvement of the aorta.

Early diagnosis and treatment are crucial for managing GCA effectively and preventing complications. If GCA is suspected, prompt referral to a specialist, such as a rheumatologist, is essential for further evaluation and management.

2.2 Treatment Options

The primary goal in treating Giant Cell Arteritis (GCA) is to reduce inflammation in the affected arteries, prevent complications such as vision loss and stroke, and manage symptoms. Treatment typically involves medications, and in some cases, lifestyle modifications and supportive therapies.

Corticosteroids

1. First-line Treatment: The cornerstone of GCA treatment is high-dose corticosteroids, such as prednisone. This medication is effective in rapidly reducing inflammation and relieving symptoms. The typical starting dose is high to ensure quick control of the disease.

2. Tapering: Once symptoms are controlled and inflammatory markers normalize, the dose of corticosteroids is gradually tapered. The tapering process can take several months to years, depending on the patient's response and the risk of relapse.

3. Monitoring: Regular monitoring of blood pressure, blood sugar, bone density, and other potential side effects is necessary due to the long-term use of corticosteroids.

Immunosuppressive Agents

1. Methotrexate: This medication is sometimes used in conjunction with corticosteroids to help reduce the dose and side effects of steroids. Methotrexate is an immunosuppressant that can be effective in maintaining remission.

2. Tocilizumab: An interleukin-6 receptor antagonist, tocilizumab has been approved for the treatment of GCA. It can be used alone or with corticosteroids and has been shown to help reduce the need for long-term steroid use.

3. Other Immunosuppressants: Drugs such as azathioprine and mycophenolate mofetil may be considered in certain cases, particularly if there is a contraindication to the use of tocilizumab or methotrexate.

Patient Education and Support

- Education: Educating patients about GCA, its treatment, and potential side effects is crucial for effective disease management. Patients should understand the importance of adhering to their medication regimen and attending regular follow-up appointments.

- Support Groups: Joining support groups or seeking counseling can provide emotional support and help patients cope with the challenges of living with a chronic illness.

The treatment of Giant Cell Arteritis involves a combination of medications, lifestyle modifications, and supportive therapies. Early and aggressive treatment is essential to control inflammation, prevent complications, and improve the quality of life for individuals with GCA.

2.3 The Importance of Nutrition in GCA Management

Nutrition plays a crucial role in managing Giant Cell Arteritis (GCA), complementing medical treatments and supporting overall health. A well-balanced diet can help reduce inflammation, manage side effects of medications, and improve quality of life. Here's a detailed look at the importance of nutrition in GCA management:

Reducing Inflammation

One of the primary goals in managing GCA is to reduce inflammation. An anti-inflammatory diet can be beneficial in this regard:

Fruits and Vegetables: Rich in antioxidants and phytonutrients, these foods help combat inflammation. Berries, leafy greens, tomatoes, and cruciferous vegetables are particularly effective.

Whole Grains: Foods like oats, quinoa, brown rice, and whole wheat provide fiber and essential nutrients that can reduce inflammation.

Healthy Fats: Omega-3 fatty acids found in fatty fish (such as salmon, mackerel, and sardines), flaxseeds, chia seeds, and walnuts have strong anti-inflammatory properties.

Lean Proteins: Chicken, turkey, tofu, and legumes are excellent sources of protein without contributing to inflammation.

Nuts and Seeds: Almonds, walnuts, flaxseeds, and chia seeds are rich in healthy fats and fiber.

Spices and Herbs: Turmeric, ginger, garlic, and cinnamon have natural anti-inflammatory effects.

Managing Side Effects of Medications

Medications used to treat GCA, particularly corticosteroids, can have side effects that may be mitigated through proper nutrition:

Bone Health: Long-term corticosteroid use can weaken bones, increasing the risk of osteoporosis.An eating regimen plentiful in calcium and vitamin D is fundamental for bone wellbeing. Dairy products, fortified plant-based milks, leafy greens, and fatty fish are good sources of these nutrients.

Blood Sugar Control: Corticosteroids can raise blood sugar levels, increasing the risk of diabetes. Limiting refined carbohydrates and sugars, and focusing on complex carbs and fiber-rich foods, can help maintain stable blood sugar levels.

Weight Management: Corticosteroids can cause weight gain and fluid retention. A balanced diet with appropriate portion sizes, combined with regular physical activity, can help manage weight.

Supporting Overall Health

Good nutrition supports overall health and can enhance the body's ability to manage GCA:

Immune Function: A diet rich in vitamins and minerals, such as vitamin C, zinc, and selenium, supports a healthy immune system. Citrus fruits, nuts, seeds, and seafood are excellent sources.

Heart Health: GCA can increase the risk of cardiovascular complications. Foods that support heart health, such as those rich in omega-3 fatty acids, fiber, and antioxidants, are beneficial.

Energy Levels: A balanced diet that includes a variety of nutrient-dense foods helps maintain energy levels and combat fatigue, a common symptom of GCA.

Nutrition is a vital component of managing Giant Cell Arteritis. By adopting an anti-inflammatory diet, managing medication side effects, and supporting overall health, individuals with GCA can improve their quality of life and enhance the effectiveness of their medical treatments.

Nutrition Basics for Giant Cell Arteritis

3.1 Anti-inflammatory Foods

A diet rich in anti-inflammatory foods can play a crucial role in managing chronic inflammatory conditions like Giant Cell Arteritis (GCA). These foods help reduce inflammation in the body, alleviate symptoms, and support overall health. Here's a detailed look at some of the most effective anti-inflammatory foods:

Fruits and Vegetables
- Berries: Blueberries, strawberries, raspberries, and blackberries are high in antioxidants called flavonoids, which reduce inflammation and protect against cellular damage.
- Leafy Greens: Spinach, kale, and Swiss chard are rich in vitamins, minerals, and antioxidants, particularly vitamin K, which has anti-inflammatory properties.
- Cruciferous Vegetables: Broccoli, cauliflower, Brussels sprouts, and cabbage contain sulforaphane, a compound that helps reduce inflammation.
- Tomatoes: Rich in lycopene, an antioxidant that reduces inflammation, especially in the lungs and throughout the body.
- Bell Peppers: Contain antioxidants like quercetin, which help reduce inflammation and oxidative stress.
- Beets: High in fiber, vitamin C, and betalains, which have anti-inflammatory and antioxidant properties.

Whole Grains
- Oats: A good source of fiber and antioxidants, oats help reduce inflammation and improve digestive health.
- Quinoa: Packed with protein, fiber, and essential nutrients, quinoa is a great anti-inflammatory grain.

- Brown Rice: Contains fiber and essential minerals that support overall health and reduce inflammation.
- Barley: High in fiber and antioxidants, barley helps reduce inflammation and supports digestive health.

Healthy Fats
- Fatty Fish: Salmon, mackerel, sardines, and trout are rich in omega-3 fatty acids, which are powerful anti-inflammatory agents.
- Olive Oil: Extra virgin olive oil contains oleocanthal, a compound with anti-inflammatory properties similar to ibuprofen.
- Avocados: Rich in monounsaturated fats, fiber, and antioxidants, avocados help reduce inflammation and support heart health.
- Nuts and Seeds: Almonds, walnuts, flaxseeds, chia seeds, and hemp seeds are high in healthy fats, fiber, and antioxidants, all of which help reduce inflammation.

Lean Proteins
- Poultry: Chicken and turkey are good sources of lean protein, which is essential for muscle repair and overall health without contributing to inflammation.
- Legumes: Beans, lentils, and chickpeas are excellent sources of plant-based protein and fiber, which help reduce inflammation and support digestive health.
- Tofu and Tempeh: Soy-based proteins that provide essential amino acids and have anti-inflammatory properties.

Spices and Herbs
- Turmeric: Contains curcumin, a potent anti-inflammatory compound. Adding black pepper to turmeric enhances the absorption of curcumin.
- Ginger: Has powerful anti-inflammatory and antioxidant effects. It can be used fresh, dried, or as a supplement.
- Garlic: Contains sulfur compounds that have anti-inflammatory effects. It can be used in a variety of dishes for flavor and health benefits.
- Cinnamon: Contains cinnamaldehyde, which has anti-inflammatory and antioxidant properties.

- Rosemary: Rich in antioxidants, rosemary helps reduce inflammation and support overall health.

Beverages
- Green Tea: Contains polyphenols, particularly epigallocatechin gallate (EGCG), which have strong anti-inflammatory and antioxidant effects.
- Herbal Teas: Teas made from turmeric, ginger, and chamomile can help reduce inflammation and support overall health.

Other Anti-inflammatory Foods
- Dark Chocolate: Rich in flavonoids, dark chocolate with a high cocoa content (70% or higher) has anti-inflammatory properties.
- Red Wine: In moderation, red wine contains resveratrol, an antioxidant that can help reduce inflammation.
- Fermented Foods: Yogurt, kefir, sauerkraut, kimchi, and other fermented foods contain probiotics, which support gut health and reduce inflammation.

Incorporating Anti-inflammatory Foods into Your Diet
- Balanced Meals: Aim to include a variety of anti-inflammatory foods in each meal. A balanced plate might include a serving of fatty fish, a generous portion of leafy greens, and a side of whole grains.
- Snacking: Choose anti-inflammatory snacks like berries, nuts, and dark chocolate.
- Cooking Methods: Opt for healthy cooking methods like steaming, grilling, roasting, and sautéing with olive oil to preserve the nutrients in your foods.
- Spices: Add spices like turmeric, ginger, and garlic to your meals for added flavor and anti-inflammatory benefits.
- Hydration: Drink plenty of water and include herbal teas to stay hydrated and support overall health.

Incorporating these anti-inflammatory foods into your diet can help manage inflammation, support overall health, and complement the treatment of Giant Cell

Arteritis. Making mindful dietary choices is a powerful tool in maintaining a healthy, balanced lifestyle.

3.2 Foods to Avoid

For individuals managing Giant Cell Arteritis (GCA), it is essential to avoid certain foods that can exacerbate inflammation and contribute to overall poor health. Eliminating or significantly reducing these foods from your diet can help manage symptoms, reduce inflammation, and support better overall health. Here's a detailed look at foods to avoid:

Processed and Refined Foods
- Refined Carbohydrates: White bread, pasta, pastries, and other refined carbohydrate products can spike blood sugar levels and increase inflammation.
- Processed Snacks: Chips, crackers, and other packaged snacks often contain unhealthy fats, sugars, and additives that promote inflammation.
- Sugary Foods and Beverages: Sodas, sweetened coffee drinks, candy, and desserts are high in sugar, which can lead to increased inflammation and contribute to weight gain and other health issues.

Red and Processed Meats
- Red Meat: Beef, lamb, and pork, especially in large quantities, can contribute to inflammation due to their high saturated fat content.
- Processed Meats: Bacon, sausage, hot dogs, and deli meats often contain high levels of preservatives, sodium, and unhealthy fats, which can increase inflammation.

Trans Fats
- Hydrogenated Oils: Found in many fried foods, baked goods, and margarines, trans fats are highly inflammatory and should be avoided.
- Commercial Baked Goods: Products like cookies, cakes, and pastries often contain trans fats and should be limited or avoided.

Excessive Alcohol
- Alcoholic Beverages: Drinking too much alcohol can lead to increased inflammation and a weakened immune system. Moderation is key, with

recommendations generally suggesting no more than one drink per day for women and two for men.

High-Sodium Foods

- Processed Foods: Many canned soups, frozen dinners, and packaged foods contain high levels of sodium, which can contribute to inflammation and high blood pressure.
- Fast Food: Often high in sodium, unhealthy fats, and calories, fast food can exacerbate inflammation and other health issues.

High-Sugar Foods

- Sugary Snacks and Desserts: Foods like candy, cookies, cakes, and ice cream are high in sugar, which can increase inflammation and contribute to weight gain and metabolic issues.
- Sweetened Beverages: Sodas, fruit juices with added sugar, energy drinks, and sweetened teas contribute to inflammation and should be avoided.

High-Fat Dairy Products

- Full-Fat Dairy: Whole milk, butter, cheese, and other high-fat dairy products contain saturated fats that can increase inflammation. Decide on low-fat or non-fat choices all things being equal.

Fried Foods

- Deep-Fried Foods: French fries, fried chicken, and other deep-fried foods are often cooked in unhealthy oils that can increase inflammation. Baking, barbecuing, or steaming are better cooking strategies.

Artificial Additives and Preservatives

- Artificial Sweeteners: Some artificial sweeteners can contribute to inflammation and other health issues. Natural sweeteners like honey or maple syrup, used in moderation, are better alternatives.
- Additives and Preservatives: Many processed foods contain additives and preservatives that can trigger inflammation. Reading labels and choosing whole, unprocessed foods is recommended.

Excessive Caffeine

- High-Caffeine Beverages: While moderate caffeine intake can have some health benefits, excessive consumption of coffee, energy drinks, and caffeinated sodas can lead to increased inflammation and other health issues.

Gluten and Dairy (for those with sensitivities)

- Gluten: For individuals with gluten sensitivity or celiac disease, gluten-containing foods such as wheat, barley, and rye can cause significant inflammation and should be avoided.

- Dairy: Those with lactose intolerance or dairy sensitivities should avoid dairy products to prevent inflammation and digestive issues.

Practical Tips for Avoiding Inflammatory Foods

- Read Labels: Pay attention to ingredient lists and nutrition labels to avoid hidden sugars, unhealthy fats, and artificial additives.

- Cook at Home: Preparing meals at home allows you to control the ingredients and avoid unhealthy additives commonly found in restaurant and processed foods.

- Choose Whole Foods: Opt for whole, unprocessed foods like fruits, vegetables, lean proteins, and whole grains to reduce inflammation and support overall health.

- Stay Hydrated: Drink plenty of water throughout the day to help flush out toxins and support bodily functions. Avoid sugary drinks and excessive alcohol.

- Plan Ahead: Plan meals and snacks in advance to ensure you have healthy options available and reduce the temptation to choose unhealthy, processed foods.

By avoiding these inflammatory foods and focusing on a balanced, nutrient-rich diet, individuals with Giant Cell Arteritis can better manage their symptoms, reduce inflammation, and improve their overall health and well-being.

3.3 Nutritional Supplements and Their Role

Nutritional supplements can play a significant role in managing Giant Cell Arteritis (GCA), supporting overall health, and addressing specific deficiencies or needs that may arise due to the condition or its treatment. While a balanced diet is the cornerstone of good nutrition, supplements can help ensure adequate intake of essential nutrients. Here's a detailed look at various supplements and their roles in GCA management:

Calcium and Vitamin D
Calcium

- Importance: Calcium is crucial for bone health, and maintaining adequate levels is essential, especially for individuals on long-term corticosteroid therapy, which can weaken bones.
- Sources: While dairy products are rich in calcium, supplements can help meet daily requirements if dietary intake is insufficient.

Vitamin D

- Importance: Vitamin D enhances calcium absorption and plays a vital role in bone health and immune function.
- Sources: Sun exposure and certain foods provide vitamin D, but supplements are often necessary to achieve optimal levels, especially in individuals with limited sun exposure or dietary intake.

Omega-3 Fatty Acids
Fish Oil Supplements

- Importance: Omega-3 fatty acids, particularly EPA and DHA, have potent anti-inflammatory properties. They can help reduce inflammation and may benefit those with GCA.

- Sources: Fatty fish like salmon, mackerel, and sardines are excellent sources, but supplements can ensure consistent intake.

Antioxidants
Vitamin C and Vitamin E

- Importance: These vitamins have antioxidant properties that help combat oxidative stress and inflammation.
- Sources: Fruits, vegetables, nuts, and seeds provide these vitamins, but supplements can be used to ensure adequate intake.

Selenium

- Importance: Selenium is a trace mineral with antioxidant properties that supports immune function and reduces inflammation.
- Sources: Brazil nuts, seafood, and meats are good dietary sources, but supplements can help meet daily needs.

B Vitamins
Vitamin B6, B12, and Folate

- Importance: These vitamins are essential for red blood cell production, nerve function, and reducing levels of homocysteine, an inflammatory marker.
- Sources: Animal products, leafy greens, and fortified foods provide these vitamins, but supplements may be necessary, particularly for individuals with dietary restrictions.

Probiotics
Probiotic Supplements

- Importance: Probiotics support gut health by maintaining a healthy balance of gut bacteria, which can influence inflammation and overall health.
- Sources: Fermented foods like yogurt, kefir, sauerkraut, and kimchi provide probiotics, but supplements can help achieve higher and more consistent intake.

Magnesium

Magnesium Supplements

- Importance: Magnesium is involved in over 300 biochemical reactions in the body, including muscle and nerve function, and it has anti-inflammatory properties.
- Sources: Leafy greens, nuts, seeds, and whole grains are dietary sources, but supplements can help meet daily requirements.

Curcumin

Turmeric/Curcumin Supplements

- Importance: Curcumin, the active compound in turmeric, has strong anti-inflammatory and antioxidant properties. It can help reduce inflammation in GCA.
- Sources: Turmeric spice provides curcumin, but supplements ensure higher and more consistent intake.

Coenzyme Q10 (CoQ10)

CoQ10 Supplements

- Importance: CoQ10 is an antioxidant that supports energy production and reduces oxidative stress and inflammation.
- Sources: Meat, fish, and whole grains provide CoQ10, but supplements can help achieve higher levels.

Practical Considerations for Supplement Use

- Consultation with Healthcare Providers: Before starting any supplement, it's crucial to consult with healthcare providers to ensure safety, especially when taking other medications or managing chronic conditions.
- Quality and Dosage: Choose high-quality supplements from reputable brands, and follow recommended dosages. Unreasonable admission of specific enhancements can make unfavorable impacts.

- Individual Needs: Supplement needs vary based on individual health status, dietary intake, and specific deficiencies. Personalized recommendations from healthcare providers are essential.
- Balanced Diet: Supplements should complement, not replace, a balanced diet rich in whole foods. A varied diet provides a wide range of nutrients that work synergistically for optimal health.
- Monitoring and Adjustment: Regular monitoring of nutrient levels through blood tests can help adjust supplement intake as needed, ensuring optimal health benefits without over-supplementation.

Nutritional supplements can play a supportive role in managing Giant Cell Arteritis by addressing specific nutrient needs, reducing inflammation, and supporting overall health. When used appropriately and in conjunction with a balanced diet, supplements can help enhance the effectiveness of medical treatments and improve quality of life for individuals with GCA.

Meal Planning and Preparation

4.1 Meal Planning Tips

Effective meal planning is essential for managing Giant Cell Arteritis (GCA) and supporting overall health. By organizing your meals in advance, you can ensure a balanced intake of nutrients, avoid inflammatory foods, and make healthier choices consistently. Here are some practical meal planning tips to help you get started:

Understand Your Nutritional Needs

- Balance Nutrients: Guarantee that every feast incorporates an equilibrium of protein, sound fats, and starches. This helps maintain energy levels and supports overall health.
- Anti-inflammatory Focus: Prioritize anti-inflammatory foods such as fruits, vegetables, whole grains, lean proteins, and healthy fats.
- Portion Control: Pay attention to portion sizes to avoid overeating and manage weight effectively.

Plan Ahead

- Weekly Planning: Set aside time each week to plan your meals. This helps streamline grocery shopping and ensures you have all the ingredients you need.
- Make a Schedule: Create a weekly meal schedule that includes breakfast, lunch, dinner, and snacks. This helps you stay organized and reduces the likelihood of last-minute unhealthy choices.
- Use a Template: Consider using a meal planning template or app to simplify the process and keep track of your plans.

Diversify Your Meals

- Variety is Key: Ensure your meal plan includes a variety of foods to provide a broad spectrum of nutrients and prevent boredom.

- Experiment with Recipes: Try new recipes and cooking techniques to keep meals interesting and enjoyable. This can also help you discover new favorite foods that fit within your dietary needs.
- Themed Nights: Consider incorporating themed nights (e.g., Meatless Monday, Taco Tuesday) to add variety and make meal planning more fun.

Prioritize Fresh and Whole Foods

- Seasonal Produce: Choose seasonal fruits and vegetables for better taste, higher nutritional value, and cost savings.
- Minimize Processed Foods: Focus on whole, unprocessed foods to reduce intake of added sugars, unhealthy fats, and preservatives.
- Healthy Substitutes: Find healthy substitutes for common ingredients. For example, use Greek yogurt instead of sour cream, or whole grain bread instead of white bread.

Stay Flexible

- Adapt as Needed: Be flexible and willing to adjust your meal plan based on changes in schedule, availability of ingredients, or personal preferences.
- Backup Meals: Have a few quick and easy backup meals or snacks ready for days when plans change or time is limited. Frozen vegetables, canned beans, and whole grain pasta can be lifesavers.
- Listen to Your Body: Pay attention to how your body responds to different foods and adjust your meal plan accordingly to support optimal health and well-being.

Involve Family and Friends

- Collaborate on Planning: Involve family members in meal planning to ensure everyone's preferences and needs are considered.
- Cooking Together: Cook meals together as a family to share responsibilities and enjoy quality time.
- Share Ideas: Exchange meal ideas and recipes with friends who have similar dietary goals or restrictions.

Monitor and Adjust

- Track Progress: Keep a food journal or use an app to track your meals and how you feel after eating. This can help identify any foods that may trigger symptoms or negatively impact your health.
- Evaluate and Adjust: Regularly review your meal plan to see what's working and what needs adjustment. This helps you stay on track with your nutritional goals and ensures you're meeting your needs.

By implementing these meal planning tips, you can create a structured, nutritious eating plan that supports the management of Giant Cell Arteritis, reduces inflammation, and promotes overall health. Effective meal planning helps you make informed choices, saves time and money, and ensures you consistently consume a balanced, anti-inflammatory diet.

4.2 Grocery Shopping Guide

Grocery shopping can be an overwhelming task, especially when trying to manage a condition like Giant Cell Arteritis (GCA) that requires careful attention to diet. This grocery shopping guide will help you navigate the aisles, make healthier choices, and ensure you have the right ingredients to support an anti-inflammatory diet.

Plan Ahead

- Create a List: Before heading to the store, plan your meals for the week and make a detailed shopping list. This helps you stay organized and focused, reducing the likelihood of impulse purchases.
- Check Your Pantry: Take inventory of what you already have at home to avoid buying duplicates and to use up existing ingredients.
- Meal Prep: Consider what ingredients can be prepared in bulk to save time during the week. Plan to buy these items in larger quantities.

Shop the Perimeter

- Fresh Produce: Spend most of your time in the produce section, which typically lines the perimeter of the store. Fill your cart with a variety of colorful fruits and vegetables, focusing on those with anti-inflammatory properties like leafy greens, berries, tomatoes, and cruciferous vegetables.
- Lean Proteins: Look for fresh, lean proteins such as chicken, turkey, fish, and plant-based options like tofu and legumes.
- Dairy Alternatives: If you need dairy products, opt for low-fat or non-fat versions. Consider alternatives like almond milk, soy milk, or oat milk if you have dairy sensitivities.

Choose Whole Grains

- Whole Grains: Opt for whole grains instead of refined grains. Look for items like quinoa, brown rice, oats, barley, and whole wheat products.

- Read Labels: Ensure that the products you choose are truly whole grain by checking the ingredient list. The first ingredient should be a whole grain (e.g., "whole wheat flour" instead of just "wheat flour").

Avoid Processed Foods

- Minimize Packaged Snacks: Stay away from the middle aisles where processed and packaged foods are typically found. These often contain added sugars, unhealthy fats, and preservatives that can increase inflammation.
- Healthy Alternatives: If you do need snacks, look for healthier options like nuts, seeds, and dried fruits without added sugars or preservatives.

Select Healthy Fats

- Olive Oil: Choose extra virgin olive oil for cooking and dressings due to its anti-inflammatory properties.
- Avocados: Include avocados in your cart for a source of healthy monounsaturated fats.
- Nuts and Seeds: Stock up on a variety of nuts and seeds like almonds, walnuts, flaxseeds, and chia seeds for snacks and recipe additions.

Smart Protein Choices

- Fish and Seafood: Aim to include fatty fish like salmon, mackerel, and sardines, which are rich in omega-3 fatty acids.
- Lean Meats: Choose lean cuts of meat and skinless poultry to reduce saturated fat intake.
- Plant-Based Proteins: Incorporate beans, lentils, chickpeas, and other legumes as excellent sources of protein and fiber.

Dairy and Dairy Alternatives

- Low-Fat Dairy: If you consume dairy, opt for low-fat or non-fat options to reduce saturated fat intake.
- Fortified Alternatives: Choose fortified plant-based milks like almond, soy, or oat milk to ensure you're getting enough calcium and vitamin D.

Frozen and Canned Options

- Frozen Fruits and Vegetables: These can be a convenient and nutritious option, especially when fresh produce is not available. Look for those without added sugars or sauces.
- Canned Beans and Tomatoes: Choose low-sodium options and rinse canned beans to reduce sodium content.

Reading Labels

- Ingredients List: The fewer ingredients, the better. Avoid products with long lists of unrecognizable ingredients.
- Nutritional Information: Pay attention to serving sizes, calories, fat content, sodium levels, and added sugars. Aim for products low in saturated fat, sodium, and added sugars.

Specialty Sections

- Organic Produce: If possible, choose organic fruits and vegetables, especially for items on the Dirty Dozen list, which are known to have higher pesticide residues.
- Gluten-Free Section: If you have gluten sensitivity or celiac disease, shop in the gluten-free section for appropriate alternatives.

Budget-Friendly Tips

- Seasonal Produce: Buy fruits and vegetables that are in season, as they are often cheaper and more flavorful.
- Bulk Bins: Purchase grains, nuts, and seeds from bulk bins to save money and reduce packaging waste.
- Store Brands: Consider store-brand items, which can be just as nutritious but less expensive than name brands.

Shopping Mindfully

- Stick to Your List: Avoid unnecessary purchases by sticking to your grocery list.
- Shop When Full: Don't shop on an empty stomach to reduce the temptation to buy unhealthy snacks.
- Stay Hydrated: Drink plenty of water while shopping to maintain energy and focus.

By following this grocery shopping guide, you can make informed decisions that support a diet designed to manage Giant Cell Arteritis, reduce inflammation, and promote overall health. Making thoughtful choices in the grocery store sets the foundation for a nutritious and balanced diet.

4.3 Batch Cooking and Meal Prep Strategies

Batch cooking and meal prep are powerful strategies to maintain a healthy diet, save time during busy weeks, and ensure you have nutritious meals ready to support the management of Giant Cell Arteritis (GCA). By preparing meals in advance, you can reduce the stress of daily cooking and make it easier to stick to an anti-inflammatory diet. Here are some effective batch cooking and meal prep strategies:

Benefits of Batch Cooking and Meal Prep

- Time-Saving: Spend less time cooking during the week by preparing meals in large quantities.
- Convenience: Have ready-to-eat meals and snacks available, making it easier to make healthy choices.
- Cost-Effective: Buying ingredients in bulk and preparing meals at home can save money compared to eating out.
- Portion Control: Control portion sizes and manage calorie intake more effectively.
- Consistency: Ensure you stick to your dietary plan and avoid last-minute unhealthy food choices.

Getting Started with Batch Cooking

- Plan Your Menu: Decide on the meals and snacks you want to prepare for the week. Aim for a mix of proteins, vegetables, whole grains, and healthy fats.
- Create a Shopping List: Make a detailed grocery list based on your menu plan to ensure you have all the necessary ingredients.
- Set Aside Time: Dedicate a specific day or time for batch cooking. Weekends are often ideal for meal prep sessions.

Essential Tools for Batch Cooking

- Quality Containers: Invest in a variety of airtight, BPA-free containers to store prepped meals and ingredients.

- Large Cooking Equipment: Use large pots, pans, and baking sheets to cook bigger batches of food at once.
- Slow Cooker or Instant Pot: These appliances can make batch cooking easier by allowing you to cook large quantities with minimal effort.

Batch Cooking Strategies

- Cook Staple Ingredients: Prepare large batches of staple ingredients like grains (quinoa, brown rice), proteins (chicken, beans), and vegetables (roasted or steamed) that can be used in various dishes throughout the week.
- Double Recipes: When cooking meals, double the recipe to have extra portions for future meals. Freeze half for later use.
- One-Pot Meals: Prepare one-pot meals like soups, stews, and casseroles that can be easily portioned and stored.
- Sheet Pan Dinners: Roast a variety of vegetables and proteins on a sheet pan for easy and efficient batch cooking.

Meal Prep Tips

- Chop and Prep Ingredients: Chop vegetables, marinate proteins, and portion out snacks ahead of time to make daily meal assembly quicker.
- Pre-Portion Meals: Divide meals into individual portions to grab and go throughout the week.
- Label and Date: Label containers with the meal name and date to keep track of freshness and reduce food waste.
- Store Properly: Use glass containers for better storage, and consider vacuum-sealing to extend the shelf life of prepped meals.

Sample Batch Cooking Plan
Proteins:

- Grilled Chicken Breasts: Season and grill chicken breasts, then slice and store for salads, wraps, or main dishes.
- Black Beans: Cook a large pot of black beans to use in tacos, grain bowls, and soups.

Vegetables:

- Roasted Vegetables: Roast a variety of vegetables like sweet potatoes, carrots, bell peppers, and broccoli with olive oil and herbs.
- Salad Greens: Wash and chop greens like kale and spinach, then store in airtight containers for quick salads.

Grains:

- Quinoa: Cook a large batch of quinoa to use as a base for grain bowls, salads, and side dishes.
- Brown Rice: Prepare brown rice to accompany proteins and vegetables in balanced meals.

Snacks:

- Hummus: Make a large batch of hummus and portion into small containers for easy snacking with veggie sticks.
- Energy Balls: Prepare no-bake energy balls with oats, nut butter, and dried fruits for quick, nutritious snacks.

Breakfast:

- Overnight Oats: Prepare jars of overnight oats with different toppings like berries, nuts, and seeds.
- Smoothie Packs: Portion out ingredients for smoothies (fruits, greens, seeds) into freezer bags for quick blending in the morning.

Freezing and Storing Meals

- Cool Before Freezing: Let hot foods cool completely before freezing to prevent ice crystals and preserve texture.
- Freeze Flat: Freeze soups, stews, and sauces flat in zip-top bags to save space and make thawing easier.

- Vacuum Seal: Use a vacuum sealer to extend the shelf life of frozen meals and prevent freezer burn.
- Reheat Properly: Thaw frozen meals in the refrigerator overnight and reheat thoroughly on the stove or in the microwave.

Staying Organized

- Weekly Review: Review your meal plan and inventory each week to ensure you have everything you need and adjust as necessary.
- Rotate Meals: Regularly rotate the meals you batch cook to keep things interesting and ensure a variety of nutrients in your diet.
- Involve Family: Get family members involved in meal prep to share the workload and make it a fun, collaborative activity.

By incorporating these batch cooking and meal prep strategies into your routine, you can simplify the process of maintaining a healthy, anti-inflammatory diet that supports the management of Giant Cell Arteritis. These practices will help you save time, reduce stress, and consistently enjoy nutritious meals throughout the week.

Breakfast Recipes

5.1 Anti-inflammatory Smoothies

1. Berry Turmeric Smoothie
Ingredients:

- 1 cup mixed berries (blueberries, strawberries, raspberries)
- 1 cup unsweetened almond milk
- 1 banana
- 1 tablespoon chia seeds
- 1 teaspoon ground turmeric
- 1 teaspoon honey or maple syrup (optional)
- 1/2 teaspoon ground cinnamon
- 1/2 teaspoon fresh ginger, grated
- 1/2 cup Greek yogurt (optional for added protein)

Directions:

1. Add all the ingredients to a blender.
2. Blend on high until smooth and creamy.
3. Taste and add honey or maple syrup if more sweetness is desired.
4. Pour into a glass and serve immediately.

Serving: 1 large or 2 small smoothies

Nutrition (per serving):

Calories: 250

Protein: 8g

Fat: 6g

Carbohydrates: 45g

Fiber: 10g

Sugar: 22g

2. Green Avocado Smoothie

Ingredients:

- 1 ripe avocado
- 1 cup spinach leaves
- 1 green apple, cored and chopped
- 1/2 cucumber, peeled and chopped
- 1 cup coconut water
- 1 tablespoon flaxseeds
- 1 tablespoon fresh lemon juice
- 1 teaspoon honey or agave nectar (optional)
- Ice cubes (optional)

Directions:

1. Add all the ingredients to a blender.
2. Blend on high until smooth and creamy.
3. Taste and add honey or agave nectar if more sweetness is desired.
4. Add ice cubes if you prefer a colder smoothie.
5. Pour into a glass and serve immediately.

Serving: 1 large or 2 small smoothies

Nutrition (per serving):

Calories: 210

Protein: 3g

Fat: 14g

Carbohydrates: 23g

Fiber: 10g

Sugar: 12g

3. Pineapple Ginger Smoothie

Ingredients:

- 1 cup pineapple chunks (fresh or frozen)
- 1 banana
- 1/2 cup unsweetened coconut milk
- 1/2 cup plain Greek yogurt
- 1 tablespoon fresh ginger, grated
- 1 tablespoon ground flaxseeds or chia seeds
- 1 teaspoon honey or maple syrup (optional)
- Ice cubes (optional)

Directions:

1. Add all the ingredients to a blender.
2. Blend on high until smooth and creamy.
3. Taste and add honey or maple syrup if more sweetness is desired.
4. Add ice cubes if you prefer a colder smoothie.
5. Pour into a glass and serve immediately.

Serving: 1 large or 2 small smoothies

Nutrition (per serving):

Calories: 260

Protein: 7g

Fat: 8g

Carbohydrates: 42g

Fiber: 6g
Sugar: 28g

4. Mango Turmeric Smoothie

Ingredients:

- 1 cup frozen mango chunks
- 1/2 cup plain Greek yogurt
- 1/2 cup coconut water or almond milk
- 1 tablespoon fresh lime juice
- 1 teaspoon ground turmeric
- 1/2 teaspoon ground ginger
- 1 tablespoon chia seeds
- Ice cubes (optional)

Directions:

1. Combine all ingredients in a blender.
2. Blend on high until smooth and creamy.
3. Add ice cubes if desired for a colder smoothie.
4. Taste and adjust sweetness or tanginess with additional lime juice or a touch of honey, if needed.
5. Pour into glasses and serve immediately.

Serving: 1 large or 2 small smoothies

Nutrition (per serving):

Calories: 240
Protein: 12g
Fat: 6g
Carbohydrates: 40g

Fiber: 7g
Sugar: 28g

5. Blueberry Spinach Smoothie

Ingredients:

- 1 cup fresh or frozen blueberries
- 1 cup spinach leaves
- 1/2 cup plain Greek yogurt
- 1 tablespoon almond butter or flaxseed meal
- 1 tablespoon honey or maple syrup
- 1/2 teaspoon vanilla extract
- 1 cup unsweetened almond milk
- Ice cubes (optional)

Directions:

1. Place all ingredients in a blender.
2. Blend until smooth and creamy.
3. Add more almond milk if needed to reach desired consistency.
4. Taste and adjust sweetness with honey or maple syrup, if desired.
5. Add ice cubes for a colder smoothie, if preferred.
6. Pour into glasses and serve immediately.

Serving: 1 large or 2 small smoothies

Nutrition (per serving):

Calories: 280
Protein: 14g
Fat: 8g
Carbohydrates: 42g

Fiber: 7g
Sugar: 28g

5.2 Nutritious Breakfast Bowls

1. Quinoa and Berry Breakfast Bowl

Ingredients:

- 1 cup cooked quinoa
- 1/2 cup mixed berries (blueberries, strawberries, raspberries)
- 1/2 banana, sliced
- 1 tablespoon chia seeds
- 1 tablespoon almond butter
- 1/2 cup unsweetened almond milk
- 1 teaspoon honey or maple syrup (optional)

Directions:

1. Place the cooked quinoa in a bowl.
2. Top with mixed berries, sliced banana, chia seeds, and almond butter.
3. Drizzle with almond milk and honey or maple syrup, if using.
4. Mix gently and serve immediately.

Serving: 1 large bowl

Nutrition (per serving):

Calories: 380

Protein: 10g

Fat: 14g

Carbohydrates: 56g

Fiber: 10g

Sugar: 16g

2. Avocado and Egg Breakfast Bowl

Ingredients:

- 1/2 avocado, sliced
- 2 eggs, poached or boiled
- 1/2 cup cherry tomatoes, halved
- 1/2 cup spinach leaves
- 1 tablespoon feta cheese, crumbled
- 1 teaspoon olive oil
- Salt and pepper to taste
- 1 slice whole grain toast (optional)

Directions:

1. Arrange the spinach leaves in a bowl.
2. Top with sliced avocado, poached or boiled eggs, cherry tomatoes, and feta cheese.
3. Drizzle with olive oil and season with salt and pepper.
4. Serve with a slice of whole grain toast, if desired.

Serving: 1 large bowl

Nutrition (per serving):

Calories: 320

Protein: 16g

Fat: 24g

Carbohydrates: 14g

Fiber: 8g

Sugar: 3g

3. Greek Yogurt and Granola Breakfast Bowl

Ingredients:

- 1 cup plain Greek yogurt
- 1/2 cup granola (preferably low-sugar)
- 1/2 cup fresh or frozen berries
- 1 tablespoon flaxseeds
- 1 tablespoon honey
- 1 tablespoon chopped nuts (almonds, walnuts, or pecans)

Directions:

1. Spoon the Greek yogurt into a bowl.
2. Top with granola, berries, flaxseeds, honey, and chopped nuts.
3. Mix gently and serve immediately.

Serving: 1 large bowl

Nutrition (per serving):

Calories: 450

Protein: 20g

Fat: 18g

Carbohydrates: 55g

Fiber: 8g

Sugar: 24g

4. Savory Oatmeal Breakfast Bowl

Ingredients:

- 1 cup cooked steel-cut oats
- 1/2 avocado, sliced

- 1 egg, poached or fried
- 1/4 cup shredded carrots
- 1/4 cup sliced cucumber
- 1 tablespoon pumpkin seeds
- 1 teaspoon soy sauce or tamari
- 1 teaspoon sesame oil
- Salt and pepper to taste

Directions:

1. Place the cooked oats in a bowl.
2. Top with sliced avocado, poached or fried egg, shredded carrots, cucumber, and pumpkin seeds.
3. Drizzle with soy sauce and sesame oil, then season with salt and pepper.
4. Mix gently and serve immediately.

Serving: 1 large bowl

Nutrition (per serving):

Calories: 400
Protein: 14g
Fat: 20g
Carbohydrates: 42g
Fiber: 10g
Sugar: 4g

5. Smoothie Bowl

Ingredients:

- 1 banana, frozen
- 1/2 cup frozen berries (blueberries, strawberries, raspberries)

- 1/2 cup spinach leaves
- 1/2 cup unsweetened almond milk
- 1 tablespoon chia seeds
- 1/4 cup granola
- 1 tablespoon coconut flakes
- 1 tablespoon almond butter

Directions:

1. In a blender, combine the frozen banana, frozen berries, spinach leaves, and almond milk. Blend until smooth.
2. Pour the smoothie into a bowl.
3. Top with chia seeds, granola, coconut flakes, and almond butter.
4. Mix gently and serve immediately.

Serving: 1 large bowl

Nutrition (per serving):

Calories: 350

Protein: 8g

Fat: 14g

Carbohydrates: 50g

Fiber: 10g

Sugar: 20g

5.3 Whole Grain and Protein-packed Options

1. Oatmeal with Berries and Nuts

Ingredients:

- 1 cup rolled oats
- 2 cups water or unsweetened almond milk
- 1/2 cup mixed berries (blueberries, strawberries, raspberries)
- 1/4 cup chopped nuts (almonds, walnuts, or pecans)
- 1 tablespoon chia seeds
- 1 tablespoon honey or maple syrup
- 1/2 teaspoon cinnamon
- Pinch of salt

Directions:

1. In a pot, bring water or almond milk to a boil.
2. Add the rolled oats, reduce heat, and simmer for 5-7 minutes, stirring occasionally.
3. Once the oats are cooked, stir in the cinnamon and a pinch of salt.
4. Pour the oatmeal into a bowl and top with mixed berries, chopped nuts, chia seeds, and honey or maple syrup.
5. Mix gently and serve immediately.

Serving: 1 large bowl

Nutrition (per serving):

Calories: 450

Protein: 12g

Fat: 18g

Carbohydrates: 62g

Fiber: 10g

Sugar: 15g

2. Quinoa Breakfast Bowl with Eggs and Avocado

Ingredients:

- 1 cup cooked quinoa
- 1 avocado, sliced
- 2 eggs, scrambled or poached
- 1/2 cup cherry tomatoes, halved
- 1/4 cup black beans, drained and rinsed
- 1 tablespoon fresh cilantro, chopped
- 1 tablespoon salsa (optional)
- Salt and pepper to taste

Directions:

1. Place the cooked quinoa in a bowl.
2. Top with scrambled or poached eggs, sliced avocado, cherry tomatoes, black beans, and fresh cilantro.
3. Add salsa if desired and season with salt and pepper.
4. Mix gently and serve immediately.

Serving: 1 large bowl

Nutrition (per serving):

Calories: 520

Protein: 20g

Fat: 30g

Carbohydrates: 45g

Fiber: 12g

Sugar: 5g

3. Farro Breakfast Bowl with Spinach and Feta

Ingredients:

- 1 cup cooked farro
- 1 cup fresh spinach leaves, sautéed
- 1/4 cup crumbled feta cheese
- 1/4 cup cherry tomatoes, halved
- 1/4 cup cucumber, chopped
- 1 tablespoon olive oil
- 1 tablespoon balsamic vinegar
- Salt and pepper to taste

Directions:

1. Place the cooked farro in a bowl.
2. Top with sautéed spinach, crumbled feta cheese, cherry tomatoes, and chopped cucumber.
3. Drizzle with olive oil and balsamic vinegar.
4. Season with salt and pepper.
5. Mix gently and serve immediately.

Serving: 1 large bowl

Nutrition (per serving):

Calories: 400
Protein: 14g
Fat: 18g
Carbohydrates: 45g
Fiber: 8g

Sugar: 4g

4. Brown Rice Breakfast Bowl with Tofu and Veggies

Ingredients:

- 1 cup cooked brown rice
- 1/2 cup firm tofu, cubed
- 1/2 cup broccoli florets, steamed
- 1/2 cup bell peppers, sliced
- 1 tablespoon soy sauce or tamari
- 1 tablespoon sesame seeds
- 1 tablespoon green onions, chopped
- 1 teaspoon sesame oil
- Salt and pepper to taste

Directions:

1. Place the cooked brown rice in a bowl.
2. Top with cubed tofu, steamed broccoli, and sliced bell peppers.
3. Drizzle with soy sauce or tamari and sesame oil.
4. Sprinkle with sesame seeds and chopped green onions.
5. Season with salt and pepper.
6. Mix gently and serve immediately.

Serving: 1 large bowl

Nutrition (per serving):

Calories: 420
Protein: 16g
Fat: 14g
Carbohydrates: 58g

Fiber: 8g

Sugar: 4g

5. Barley Breakfast Bowl with Smoked Salmon

Ingredients:

- 1 cup cooked barley
- 2 oz smoked salmon
- 1/2 avocado, sliced
- 1/4 cup cucumber, chopped
- 1 tablespoon capers
- 1 tablespoon fresh dill, chopped
- 1 tablespoon lemon juice
- 1 tablespoon olive oil
- Salt and pepper to taste

Directions:

1. Place the cooked barley in a bowl.
2. Top with smoked salmon, sliced avocado, chopped cucumber, and capers.
3. Drizzle with lemon juice and olive oil.
4. Sprinkle with fresh dill.
5. Season with salt and pepper.
6. Mix gently and serve immediately.

Serving: 1 large bowl

Nutrition (per serving):

Calories: 460

Protein: 20g

Fat: 24g

Carbohydrates: 42g
Fiber: 10g
Sugar: 3g

Lunch Recipes

6.1 Salads and Grain Bowls

1. Mediterranean Quinoa Salad

Ingredients:

- 1 cup cooked quinoa
- 1/2 cup cherry tomatoes, halved
- 1/2 cup cucumber, diced
- 1/4 cup red onion, finely chopped
- 1/4 cup Kalamata olives, sliced
- 1/4 cup feta cheese, crumbled
- 1/4 cup fresh parsley, chopped
- 2 tablespoons olive oil
- 1 tablespoon lemon juice
- Salt and pepper to taste

Directions:

1. In a large bowl, combine the cooked quinoa, cherry tomatoes, cucumber, red onion, olives, feta cheese, and parsley.
2. Drizzle with olive oil and lemon juice, then season with salt and pepper.
3. Toss gently to combine.
4. Serve immediately or refrigerate until ready to eat.

Serving: 2 servings

Nutrition (per serving):

Calories: 320

Protein: 9g

Fat: 20g

Carbohydrates: 28g

Fiber: 5g

Sugar: 4g

2. Southwest Black Bean and Avocado Salad

Ingredients:

- 1 can (15 oz) black beans, drained and rinsed
- 1 cup corn kernels (fresh or frozen, thawed)
- 1 red bell pepper, diced
- 1 avocado, diced
- 1/4 cup red onion, finely chopped
- 1/4 cup fresh cilantro, chopped
- 2 tablespoons lime juice
- 1 tablespoon olive oil
- 1/2 teaspoon cumin
- Salt and pepper to taste

Directions:

1. In a large bowl, combine the black beans, corn, bell pepper, avocado, red onion, and cilantro.
2. In a small bowl, whisk together the lime juice, olive oil, cumin, salt, and pepper.
3. Pour the dressing over the salad and toss gently to combine.
4. Serve immediately or refrigerate until ready to eat.

Serving: 2 servings

Nutrition (per serving):

Calories: 360
Protein: 10g
Fat: 18g
Carbohydrates: 45g
Fiber: 15g
Sugar: 5g

3. Asian Chicken and Brown Rice Bowl
Ingredients:

- 1 cup cooked brown rice
- 1 cup cooked chicken breast, shredded
- 1 cup shredded carrots
- 1 cup sliced cucumber
- 1/4 cup edamame beans, shelled
- 2 tablespoons green onions, sliced
- 2 tablespoons sesame seeds
- 2 tablespoons soy sauce or tamari
- 1 tablespoon rice vinegar
- 1 tablespoon sesame oil
- 1 teaspoon honey
- 1 clove garlic, minced
- 1 teaspoon fresh ginger, grated

Directions:

1. In a large bowl, combine the cooked brown rice, shredded chicken, carrots, cucumber, edamame, and green onions.

2. In a small bowl, whisk together the soy sauce, rice vinegar, sesame oil, honey, garlic, and ginger.
3. Pour the dressing over the rice bowl and toss gently to combine.
4. Sprinkle with sesame seeds before serving.

Serving: 2 servings

Nutrition (per serving):

Calories: 450
Protein: 32g
Fat: 15g
Carbohydrates: 45g
Fiber: 6g
Sugar: 5g

4. Greek Chicken and Farro Bowl

Ingredients:

- 1 cup cooked farro
- 1 cup cooked chicken breast, diced
- 1/2 cup cherry tomatoes, halved
- 1/2 cup cucumber, diced
- 1/4 cup red onion, finely chopped
- 1/4 cup Kalamata olives, sliced
- 1/4 cup feta cheese, crumbled
- 1/4 cup fresh dill, chopped
- 2 tablespoons olive oil
- 1 tablespoon red wine vinegar
- Salt and pepper to taste

Directions:

1. In a large bowl, combine the cooked farro, diced chicken, cherry tomatoes, cucumber, red onion, olives, feta cheese, and dill.
2. Drizzle with olive oil and red wine vinegar, then season with salt and pepper.
3. Toss gently to combine.
4. Serve immediately or refrigerate until ready to eat.

Serving: 2 servings

Nutrition (per serving):

Calories: 410

Protein: 28g

Fat: 18g

Carbohydrates: 38g

Fiber: 7g

Sugar: 4g

5. Sweet Potato and Chickpea Bowl

Ingredients:

- 1 cup roasted sweet potato cubes
- 1 can (15 oz) chickpeas, drained and rinsed
- 1 cup cooked quinoa
- 1/2 avocado, sliced
- 1/4 cup red onion, finely chopped
- 2 tablespoons tahini
- 2 tablespoons lemon juice
- 1 tablespoon olive oil
- 1 clove garlic, minced

- Salt and pepper to taste
- Fresh parsley, chopped (optional)

Directions:

1. In a large bowl, combine the roasted sweet potato, chickpeas, cooked quinoa, avocado, and red onion.
2. In a small bowl, whisk together the tahini, lemon juice, olive oil, garlic, salt, and pepper.
3. Pour the dressing over the bowl and toss gently to combine.
4. Sprinkle with chopped parsley if desired.
5. Serve immediately or refrigerate until ready to eat.

Serving: 2 servings

Nutrition (per serving):

Calories: 430
Protein: 13g
Fat: 20g
Carbohydrates: 50g
Fiber: 12g
Sugar: 8g

6.2 Hearty Soups and Stews

1. Lentil and Vegetable Stew

Ingredients:

- 1 cup dry green or brown lentils, rinsed
- 1 tablespoon olive oil
- 1 large onion, chopped
- 3 cloves garlic, minced
- 3 carrots, diced
- 2 celery stalks, diced
- 1 zucchini, diced
- 1 can (14.5 oz) diced tomatoes
- 6 cups vegetable broth
- 1 teaspoon ground cumin
- 1 teaspoon smoked paprika
- 1/2 teaspoon dried thyme
- Salt and pepper to taste
- 2 cups fresh spinach leaves

Directions:

1. In a large pot, heat the olive oil over medium heat.
2. Add the onion and garlic, and sauté until fragrant and softened, about 5 minutes.
3. Add the carrots, celery, and zucchini, and cook for another 5 minutes.
4. Stir in the lentils, diced tomatoes, vegetable broth, cumin, smoked paprika, thyme, salt, and pepper.
5. Bring to a boil, then reduce heat and simmer for 30-35 minutes, or until the lentils are tender.
6. Stir in the spinach leaves and cook until wilted, about 2 minutes.
7. Serve hot.

Serving: 4 servings

Nutrition (per serving):

Calories: 270
Protein: 14g
Fat: 6g
Carbohydrates: 42g
Fiber: 14g
Sugar: 10g

2. Chicken and Wild Rice Soup

Ingredients:

- 1 tablespoon olive oil
- 1 medium onion, chopped
- 3 cloves garlic, minced
- 3 carrots, diced
- 2 celery stalks, diced
- 1 cup wild rice, rinsed
- 6 cups chicken broth
- 2 cups cooked chicken breast, shredded
- 1 teaspoon dried thyme
- 1 teaspoon dried rosemary
- Salt and pepper to taste
- 1 cup coconut milk (optional for creaminess)
- 2 tablespoons fresh parsley, chopped

Directions:

1. In a large pot, heat the olive oil over medium heat.

2. Add the onion and garlic, and sauté until fragrant and softened, about 5 minutes.
3. Add the carrots and celery, and cook for another 5 minutes.
4. Stir in the wild rice, chicken broth, cooked chicken, thyme, rosemary, salt, and pepper.
5. Bring to a boil, then reduce heat and simmer for 40-45 minutes, or until the wild rice is tender.
6. Stir in the coconut milk, if using, and heat through.
7. Garnish with fresh parsley before serving.

Serving: 4 servings

Nutrition (per serving):

Calories: 350
Protein: 24g
Fat: 12g
Carbohydrates: 35g
Fiber: 5g
Sugar: 5g

3. Beef and Barley Stew

Ingredients:

- 1 tablespoon olive oil
- 1 pound beef stew meat, cut into cubes
- 1 large onion, chopped
- 3 cloves garlic, minced
- 3 carrots, diced
- 2 celery stalks, diced
- 1 cup pearl barley
- 6 cups beef broth

- 1 can (14.5 oz) diced tomatoes
- 1 teaspoon dried thyme
- 1 teaspoon dried rosemary
- Salt and pepper to taste
- 2 cups baby spinach (optional)

Directions:

1. In a large pot, heat the olive oil over medium heat.
2. Add the beef cubes and brown on all sides. Remove from the pot and set aside.
3. In the same pot, add the onion and garlic, and sauté until fragrant and softened, about 5 minutes.
4. Add the carrots and celery, and cook for another 5 minutes.
5. Stir in the barley, beef broth, diced tomatoes, thyme, rosemary, salt, and pepper.
6. Return the browned beef to the pot.
7. Bring to a boil, then reduce heat and simmer for 1 hour, or until the beef and barley are tender.
8. Stir in the baby spinach, if using, and cook until wilted, about 2 minutes.
9. Serve hot.

Serving: 4 servings

Nutrition (per serving):

Calories: 400
Protein: 30g
Fat: 12g
Carbohydrates: 45g
Fiber: 8g
Sugar: 8g

4. Sweet Potato and Black Bean Soup

Ingredients:

- 1 tablespoon olive oil
- 1 large onion, chopped
- 3 cloves garlic, minced
- 2 large sweet potatoes, peeled and diced
- 1 red bell pepper, diced
- 1 can (14.5 oz) diced tomatoes
- 4 cups vegetable broth
- 1 can (15 oz) black beans, drained and rinsed
- 1 teaspoon ground cumin
- 1 teaspoon smoked paprika
- 1/2 teaspoon chili powder
- Salt and pepper to taste
- 1/4 cup fresh cilantro, chopped

Directions:

1. In a large pot, heat the olive oil over medium heat.
2. Add the onion and garlic, and sauté until fragrant and softened, about 5 minutes.
3. Add the sweet potatoes and red bell pepper, and cook for another 5 minutes.
4. Stir in the diced tomatoes, vegetable broth, black beans, cumin, smoked paprika, chili powder, salt, and pepper.
5. Bring to a boil, then reduce heat and simmer for 20-25 minutes, or until the sweet potatoes are tender.
6. Garnish with fresh cilantro before serving.

Serving: 4 servings

Nutrition (per serving):

Calories: 320

Protein: 9g

Fat: 8g

Carbohydrates: 54g

Fiber: 14g

Sugar: 12g

5. Curried Chickpea Stew

Ingredients:

- 1 tablespoon olive oil
- 1 large onion, chopped
- 3 cloves garlic, minced
- 1 tablespoon fresh ginger, grated
- 2 large carrots, diced
- 1 red bell pepper, diced
- 1 can (14.5 oz) diced tomatoes
- 1 can (15 oz) chickpeas, drained and rinsed
- 1 can (14 oz) coconut milk
- 2 cups vegetable broth
- 1 tablespoon curry powder
- 1 teaspoon ground cumin
- 1 teaspoon ground coriander
- Salt and pepper to taste
- 2 cups fresh spinach leaves
- 1/4 cup fresh cilantro, chopped

Directions:

1. In a large pot, heat the olive oil over medium heat.

2. Add the onion, garlic, and ginger, and sauté until fragrant and softened, about 5 minutes.
3. Add the carrots and red bell pepper, and cook for another 5 minutes.
4. Stir in the diced tomatoes, chickpeas, coconut milk, vegetable broth, curry powder, cumin, coriander, salt, and pepper.
5. Bring to a boil, then reduce heat and simmer for 20-25 minutes, or until the vegetables are tender.
6. Stir in the spinach leaves and cook until wilted, about 2 minutes.
7. Garnish with fresh cilantro before serving.

Serving: 4 servings

Nutrition (per serving):

Calories: 370
Protein: 10g
Fat: 20g
Carbohydrates: 45g
Fiber: 12g
Sugar: 10g

6.3 Healthy Sandwiches and Wraps

1. Mediterranean Veggie Wrap

Ingredients:

- 1 whole wheat tortilla
- 1/4 cup hummus
- 1/2 cup mixed greens
- 1/4 cup cucumber, sliced
- 1/4 cup red bell pepper, sliced
- 1/4 cup cherry tomatoes, halved
- 1/4 cup Kalamata olives, sliced
- 1/4 cup feta cheese, crumbled
- 1 tablespoon fresh parsley, chopped

Directions:

1. Lay the whole wheat tortilla flat on a clean surface.
2. Spread the hummus evenly over the tortilla.
3. Layer the mixed greens, cucumber, red bell pepper, cherry tomatoes, olives, feta cheese, and parsley on top of the hummus.
4. Roll up the tortilla tightly, tucking in the sides as you go.
5. Cut the wrap in half and serve immediately.

Serving: 1 serving

Nutrition (per serving):

Calories: 350

Protein: 10g

Fat: 18g

Carbohydrates: 40g

Fiber: 8g

Sugar: 6g

2. Grilled Chicken and Avocado Sandwich

Ingredients:

- 2 slices whole grain bread
- 1/2 avocado, mashed
- 1/2 cup cooked chicken breast, sliced
- 1/4 cup spinach leaves
- 2 slices tomato
- 1 slice red onion
- 1 tablespoon Dijon mustard

Directions:

1. Toast the whole grain bread slices until golden brown.
2. Spread the mashed avocado on one slice of the toasted bread.
3. Layer the cooked chicken, spinach leaves, tomato slices, and red onion on top of the avocado.
4. Spread the Dijon mustard on the other slice of bread and place it on top of the sandwich.
5. Cut the sandwich in half and serve immediately.

Serving: 1 serving

Nutrition (per serving):

Calories: 380

Protein: 25g

Fat: 18g

Carbohydrates: 32g

Fiber: 8g

Sugar: 4g

3. Turkey and Cranberry Wrap

Ingredients:

- 1 whole wheat tortilla
- 2 tablespoons cranberry sauce (low sugar)
- 1/2 cup sliced turkey breast
- 1/4 cup mixed greens
- 1/4 cup shredded carrots
- 1/4 cup sliced cucumber
- 1 tablespoon chopped pecans (optional)

Directions:

1. Lay the whole wheat tortilla flat on a clean surface.
2. Spread the cranberry sauce evenly over the tortilla.
3. Layer the turkey slices, mixed greens, shredded carrots, cucumber, and pecans (if using) on top of the cranberry sauce.
4. Roll up the tortilla tightly, tucking in the sides as you go.
5. Cut the wrap in half and serve immediately.

Serving: 1 serving

Nutrition (per serving):

Calories: 340

Protein: 20g

Fat: 10g

Carbohydrates: 42g

Fiber: 7g

Sugar: 10g

4. Hummus and Veggie Sandwich
Ingredients:

- 2 slices whole grain bread
- 1/4 cup hummus
- 1/4 cup shredded carrots
- 1/4 cup cucumber, sliced
- 1/4 cup red bell pepper, sliced
- 1/4 cup alfalfa sprouts
- 1/4 cup spinach leaves

Directions:

1. Toast the whole grain bread slices until golden brown.
2. Spread the hummus evenly over one slice of the toasted bread.
3. Layer the shredded carrots, cucumber slices, red bell pepper, alfalfa sprouts, and spinach leaves on top of the hummus.
4. Place the other slice of bread on top to complete the sandwich.
5. Cut the sandwich in half and serve immediately.

Serving: 1 serving

Nutrition (per serving):

Calories: 320
Protein: 10g
Fat: 12g
Carbohydrates: 44g
Fiber: 10g
Sugar: 6g

5. Tuna and Avocado Wrap

Ingredients:

- 1 whole wheat tortilla
- 1 can (5 oz) tuna, drained
- 1/2 avocado, mashed
- 1 tablespoon plain Greek yogurt
- 1 teaspoon Dijon mustard
- 1/4 cup shredded lettuce
- 1/4 cup shredded carrots
- 1/4 cup diced celery
- Salt and pepper to taste

Directions:

1. In a medium bowl, combine the tuna, mashed avocado, Greek yogurt, and Dijon mustard. Mix well.
2. Lay the whole wheat tortilla flat on a clean surface.
3. Spread the tuna mixture evenly over the tortilla.
4. Layer the shredded lettuce, shredded carrots, and diced celery on top of the tuna mixture.
5. Season with salt and pepper to taste.
6. Roll up the tortilla tightly, tucking in the sides as you go.
7. Cut the wrap in half and serve immediately.

Serving: 1 serving

Nutrition (per serving):

Calories: 360
Protein: 28g
Fat: 16g

Carbohydrates: 28g

Fiber: 7g

Sugar: 4g

Dinner Recipes

7.1 Balanced and Nutritious Main Dishes

1. Baked Salmon with Quinoa and Asparagus
Ingredients:

- 4 salmon fillets (about 6 oz each)
- 1 cup quinoa, rinsed
- 2 cups vegetable broth
- 1 bunch asparagus, trimmed
- 2 tablespoons olive oil
- 1 lemon, sliced
- 2 cloves garlic, minced
- Salt and pepper to taste
- Fresh parsley, chopped (for garnish)

Directions:

1. Preheat the oven to 400°F (200°C).
2. In a medium saucepan, bring the vegetable broth to a boil. Add the quinoa, reduce heat, cover, and simmer for 15 minutes, or until the liquid is absorbed and the quinoa is tender. Fluff with a fork.
3. While the quinoa is cooking, place the salmon fillets on a baking sheet lined with parchment paper. Arrange the asparagus around the salmon.
4. Drizzle the olive oil over the salmon and asparagus. Sprinkle with garlic, salt, and pepper.
5. Place lemon slices on top of the salmon fillets.
6. Bake in the preheated oven for 15-20 minutes, or until the salmon is cooked through and flakes easily with a fork.

7. Serve the salmon and asparagus over the cooked quinoa. Garnish with fresh parsley.

Serving: 4 servings

Nutrition (per serving):

Calories: 450

Protein: 36g

Fat: 20g

Carbohydrates: 28g

Fiber: 6g

Sugar: 2g

2. Chicken Stir-Fry with Brown Rice

Ingredients:

- 1 cup brown rice
- 2 cups water
- 2 tablespoons olive oil
- 1 pound boneless, skinless chicken breast, cut into strips
- 2 cups broccoli florets
- 1 red bell pepper, sliced
- 1 yellow bell pepper, sliced
- 1 carrot, sliced
- 3 cloves garlic, minced
- 1 tablespoon fresh ginger, grated
- 1/4 cup low-sodium soy sauce
- 1 tablespoon honey
- 1 tablespoon rice vinegar
- 1 teaspoon sesame oil

- 1 tablespoon sesame seeds (optional)
- Fresh cilantro, chopped (for garnish)

Directions:

1. In a medium saucepan, bring the water to a boil. Add the brown rice, reduce heat, cover, and simmer for 45 minutes, or until the rice is tender and the water is absorbed. Fluff with a fork.
2. While the rice is cooking, heat the olive oil in a large skillet or wok over medium-high heat.
3. Add the chicken strips and cook until browned and cooked through, about 5-7 minutes. Remove the chicken from the skillet and set aside.
4. In the same skillet, add the broccoli, bell peppers, and carrot. Cook for 5-7 minutes, or until the vegetables are tender-crisp.
5. Add the garlic and ginger, and cook for another 1-2 minutes, until fragrant.
6. In a small bowl, whisk together the soy sauce, honey, rice vinegar, and sesame oil. Pour the sauce over the vegetables and return the chicken to the skillet. Stir to coat.
7. Cook for an additional 2-3 minutes, until everything is heated through.
8. Serve the stir-fry over the cooked brown rice. Sprinkle with sesame seeds and garnish with fresh cilantro.

Serving: 4 servings

Nutrition (per serving):

Calories: 420
Protein: 30g
Fat: 12g
Carbohydrates: 48g
Fiber: 6g
Sugar: 9g

3. Quinoa Stuffed Bell Peppers

Ingredients:

- 4 large bell peppers (any color)
- 1 cup quinoa, rinsed
- 2 cups vegetable broth
- 1 tablespoon olive oil
- 1 onion, chopped
- 2 cloves garlic, minced
- 1 can (15 oz) black beans, drained and rinsed
- 1 cup corn kernels (fresh or frozen)
- 1 cup diced tomatoes
- 1 teaspoon ground cumin
- 1 teaspoon chili powder
- Salt and pepper to taste
- 1 cup shredded cheddar cheese
- Fresh cilantro, chopped (for garnish)

Directions:

1. Preheat the oven to 375°F (190°C).
2. In a medium saucepan, bring the vegetable broth to a boil. Add the quinoa, reduce heat, cover, and simmer for 15 minutes, or until the liquid is absorbed and the quinoa is tender. Fluff with a fork.
3. While the quinoa is cooking, cut the tops off the bell peppers and remove the seeds. Place the peppers in a baking dish.
4. In a large skillet, heat the olive oil over medium heat. Add the onion and garlic, and sauté until softened, about 5 minutes.

5. Stir in the cooked quinoa, black beans, corn, diced tomatoes, cumin, chili powder, salt, and pepper. Cook for an additional 5 minutes, until heated through.

6. Spoon the quinoa mixture into the bell peppers, filling them completely. Sprinkle the tops with shredded cheddar cheese.

7. Cover the baking dish with foil and bake in the preheated oven for 30 minutes. Remove the foil and bake for an additional 10 minutes, or until the peppers are tender and the cheese is melted and bubbly.

8. Garnish with fresh cilantro before serving.

Serving: 4 servings

Nutrition (per serving):

Calories: 380
Protein: 15g
Fat: 14g
Carbohydrates: 53g
Fiber: 12g
Sugar: 9g

4. Turkey Meatballs with Zucchini Noodles
Ingredients:

1. 1 pound ground turkey
2. 1/4 cup whole wheat breadcrumbs
3. 1/4 cup grated Parmesan cheese
4. 1 egg, beaten
5. 2 cloves garlic, minced
6. 1 tablespoon fresh parsley, chopped
7. Salt and pepper to taste

8. 2 tablespoons olive oil

9. 4 large zucchinis, spiralized into noodles

10. 2 cups marinara sauce (store-bought or homemade)

11. Fresh basil, chopped (for garnish)

Directions:

1. In a large bowl, combine the ground turkey, breadcrumbs, Parmesan cheese, egg, garlic, parsley, salt, and pepper. Mix until well combined.

2. Form the mixture into small meatballs, about 1 inch in diameter.

3. In a large skillet, heat the olive oil over medium-high heat. Add the meatballs and cook until browned on all sides and cooked through, about 10 minutes.

4. While the meatballs are cooking, bring a pot of water to a boil. Add the zucchini noodles and cook for 2-3 minutes, until just tender. Drain and set aside.

5. In a small saucepan, heat the marinara sauce over medium heat until warmed through.

6. Serve the meatballs over the zucchini noodles, topped with marinara sauce. Garnish with fresh basil.

Serving: 4 servings

Nutrition (per serving):

Calories: 350

Protein: 28g

Fat: 18g

Carbohydrates: 20g

Fiber: 5g

Sugar: 8g

5. Shrimp and Broccoli Stir-Fry

Ingredients:

- 2 tablespoons olive oil
- 1 pound shrimp, peeled and deveined
- 4 cups broccoli florets
- 1 red bell pepper, sliced
- 3 cloves garlic, minced
- 1 tablespoon fresh ginger, grated
- 1/4 cup low-sodium soy sauce
- 1 tablespoon honey
- 1 tablespoon rice vinegar
- 1 teaspoon sesame oil
- 1 tablespoon sesame seeds (optional)
- Fresh cilantro, chopped (for garnish)
- 2 cups cooked brown rice

Directions:

1. In a large skillet or wok, heat 1 tablespoon of olive oil over medium-high heat. Add the shrimp and cook until pink and opaque, about 2-3 minutes per side. Remove from the skillet and set aside.
2. In the same skillet, add the remaining olive oil. Add the broccoli and red bell pepper, and cook for 5-7 minutes, until the vegetables are tender-crisp.
3. Add the garlic and ginger, and cook for another 1-2 minutes, until fragrant.
4. In a small bowl, whisk together the soy sauce, honey, rice vinegar, and sesame oil. Pour the sauce over the vegetables and return the shrimp to the skillet. Stir to coat.
5. Cook for an additional 2-3 minutes, until everything is heated through.
6. Serve the stir-fry over the cooked brown rice. Sprinkle with sesame seeds and garnish with fresh cilantro.

Serving: 4 servings

Nutrition (per serving):

Calories: 380
Protein: 30g
Fat: 12g
Carbohydrates: 38g
Fiber: 6g
Sugar: 8g

7.2 Vegetable-focused Entrees

1. Stuffed Portobello Mushrooms

Ingredients:

- 4 large portobello mushrooms, stems removed
- 1 tablespoon olive oil
- 1 onion, finely chopped
- 2 cloves garlic, minced
- 1 cup spinach, chopped
- 1/2 cup cherry tomatoes, halved
- 1/2 cup breadcrumbs (whole wheat preferred)
- 1/4 cup grated Parmesan cheese
- Salt and pepper to taste
- Fresh basil, chopped (for garnish)

Directions:

1. Preheat the oven to 375°F (190°C).
2. Brush the portobello mushrooms with olive oil and place them on a baking sheet, gill side up.
3. In a skillet, heat the olive oil over medium heat. Add the onion and garlic and sauté until softened, about 5 minutes.
4. Add the spinach and cherry tomatoes to the skillet and cook until the spinach is wilted, about 3 minutes.
5. Remove from heat and stir in the breadcrumbs, Parmesan cheese, salt, and pepper.
6. Spoon the mixture evenly into the portobello mushrooms.
7. Bake in the preheated oven for 20-25 minutes, until the mushrooms are tender and the filling is golden brown.
8. Garnish with fresh basil before serving.

Serving: 4 servings

Nutrition (per serving):

Calories: 180
Protein: 7g
Fat: 10g
Carbohydrates: 18g
Fiber: 4g
Sugar: 4g

2. Ratatouille

Ingredients:

- 2 tablespoons olive oil
- 1 onion, chopped
- 3 cloves garlic, minced
- 1 eggplant, diced
- 1 zucchini, sliced
- 1 yellow squash, sliced
- 1 red bell pepper, chopped
- 1 yellow bell pepper, chopped
- 4 tomatoes, chopped
- 1 teaspoon dried thyme
- 1 teaspoon dried oregano
- Salt and pepper to taste
- Fresh basil, chopped (for garnish)

Directions:

1. In a large pot, heat the olive oil over medium heat. Add the onion and garlic and sauté until softened, about 5 minutes.
2. Add the eggplant, zucchini, yellow squash, red bell pepper, and yellow bell pepper to the pot. Cook, stirring occasionally, until the vegetables begin to soften, about 10 minutes.
3. Add the tomatoes, thyme, oregano, salt, and pepper. Stir to combine.
4. Reduce heat to low, cover, and simmer for 30 minutes, stirring occasionally, until the vegetables are tender and the flavors are well combined.
5. Serve hot, garnished with fresh basil.

Serving: 6 servings

Nutrition (per serving):

Calories: 120
Protein: 2g
Fat: 7g
Carbohydrates: 14g
Fiber: 5g
Sugar: 8g

3. Lentil and Vegetable Stew
Ingredients:

- 1 tablespoon olive oil
- 1 onion, chopped
- 2 cloves garlic, minced
- 2 carrots, sliced
- 2 celery stalks, chopped

- 1 zucchini, chopped
- 1 red bell pepper, chopped
- 1 cup lentils, rinsed
- 4 cups vegetable broth
- 1 can (14.5 oz) diced tomatoes
- 1 teaspoon dried thyme
- 1 teaspoon dried rosemary
- Salt and pepper to taste
- Fresh parsley, chopped (for garnish)

Directions:

1. In a large pot, heat the olive oil over medium heat. Add the onion and garlic and sauté until softened, about 5 minutes.
2. Add the carrots, celery, zucchini, and red bell pepper to the pot. Cook, stirring occasionally, for 5-7 minutes.
3. Add the lentils, vegetable broth, diced tomatoes, thyme, rosemary, salt, and pepper. Stir to combine.
4. Bring to a boil, then reduce heat to low. Cover and simmer for 30-40 minutes, or until the lentils and vegetables are tender.
5. Serve hot, garnished with fresh parsley.

Serving: 6 servings

Nutrition (per serving):

Calories: 200
Protein: 10g
Fat: 3g
Carbohydrates: 35g
Fiber: 12g
Sugar: 7g

4. Roasted Vegetable and Chickpea Bowl

Ingredients:

- 1 cup quinoa, rinsed
- 2 cups vegetable broth
- 1 sweet potato, diced
- 1 red bell pepper, chopped
- 1 zucchini, sliced
- 1 cup cherry tomatoes, halved
- 1 can (15 oz) chickpeas, drained and rinsed
- 2 tablespoons olive oil
- 1 teaspoon paprika
- 1 teaspoon cumin
- Salt and pepper to taste
- Fresh parsley, chopped (for garnish)
- Lemon wedges (for serving)

Directions:

1. Preheat the oven to 400°F (200°C).
2. In a medium saucepan, bring the vegetable broth to a boil. Add the quinoa, reduce heat, cover, and simmer for 15 minutes, or until the liquid is absorbed and the quinoa is tender. Fluff with a fork.
3. While the quinoa is cooking, place the sweet potato, red bell pepper, zucchini, cherry tomatoes, and chickpeas on a baking sheet. Drizzle with olive oil, and sprinkle with paprika, cumin, salt, and pepper. Toss to coat.
4. Roast in the preheated oven for 25-30 minutes, or until the vegetables are tender and slightly caramelized.
5. Divide the cooked quinoa among bowls and top with the roasted vegetables and chickpeas. Garnish with fresh parsley and serve with lemon wedges.

Serving: 4 servings

Nutrition (per serving):

Calories: 320
Protein: 10g
Fat: 12g
Carbohydrates: 46g
Fiber: 10g
Sugar: 8g

5. Cauliflower Curry

Ingredients:

- 2 tablespoons coconut oil
- 1 onion, chopped
- 3 cloves garlic, minced
- 1 tablespoon fresh ginger, grated
- 1 tablespoon curry powder
- 1 teaspoon ground turmeric
- 1 teaspoon ground cumin
- 1 head cauliflower, chopped into florets
- 1 can (14.5 oz) diced tomatoes
- 1 can (14 oz) coconut milk
- 1 cup frozen peas
- Salt and pepper to taste
- Fresh cilantro, chopped (for garnish)
- Cooked brown rice (for serving)

Directions:

1. In a large pot, heat the coconut oil over medium heat. Add the onion, garlic, and ginger, and sauté until softened, about 5 minutes.
2. Stir in the curry powder, turmeric, and cumin, and cook for 1-2 minutes, until fragrant.
3. Add the cauliflower florets, diced tomatoes, and coconut milk. Stir to combine.
4. Bring to a boil, then reduce heat to low. Cover and simmer for 20-25 minutes, or until the cauliflower is tender.
5. Stir in the frozen peas and cook for an additional 5 minutes, until heated through.
6. Season with salt and pepper to taste.
7. Serve the curry over cooked brown rice, garnished with fresh cilantro.

Serving: 6 servings

Nutrition (per serving):

Calories: 300
Protein: 6g
Fat: 18g
Carbohydrates: 32g
Fiber: 8g
Sugar: 8g

7.3 Lean Protein Options

1. Lemon Herb Grilled Chicken

Ingredients:

- 4 boneless, skinless chicken breasts
- 2 tablespoons olive oil
- 2 tablespoons lemon juice
- 1 tablespoon lemon zest
- 2 cloves garlic, minced
- 1 tablespoon fresh rosemary, chopped
- 1 tablespoon fresh thyme, chopped
- Salt and pepper to taste

Directions:

1. In a bowl, combine olive oil, lemon juice, lemon zest, garlic, rosemary, thyme, salt, and pepper.
2. Place the chicken breasts in a resealable plastic bag and pour the marinade over them. Seal the bag and marinate in the refrigerator for at least 30 minutes.
3. Preheat the grill to medium-high heat.
4. Remove the chicken from the marinade and grill for 6-8 minutes per side, or until the internal temperature reaches 165°F (74°C).
5. Let the chicken rest for 5 minutes before serving.

Serving: 4 servings

Nutrition (per serving):

Calories: 220

Protein: 30g

Fat: 10g

Carbohydrates: 1g

Fiber: 0g

Sugar: 0g

2. Baked Salmon with Dill

Ingredients:

- 4 salmon fillets (6 oz each)
- 2 tablespoons olive oil
- 1 tablespoon fresh lemon juice
- 1 tablespoon fresh dill, chopped
- 1 clove garlic, minced
- Salt and pepper to taste

Directions:

1. Preheat the oven to 375°F (190°C).
2. In a small bowl, combine olive oil, lemon juice, dill, garlic, salt, and pepper.
3. Place the salmon fillets on a baking sheet lined with parchment paper.
4. Brush the salmon with the olive oil mixture.
5. Bake for 15-20 minutes, or until the salmon flakes easily with a fork.
6. Serve with a side of steamed vegetables or a salad.

Serving: 4 servings

Nutrition (per serving):

Calories: 310

Protein: 34g

Fat: 18g

Carbohydrates: 1g

Fiber: 0g

Sugar: 0g

3. Turkey and Vegetable Stir-fry

Ingredients:

- 1 lb ground turkey (93% lean)
- 2 tablespoons olive oil
- 1 onion, sliced
- 2 cloves garlic, minced
- 1 red bell pepper, sliced
- 1 yellow bell pepper, sliced
- 1 zucchini, sliced
- 2 cups broccoli florets
- 2 tablespoons low-sodium soy sauce
- 1 tablespoon hoisin sauce
- 1 teaspoon fresh ginger, grated
- Salt and pepper to taste
- Cooked brown rice (for serving)

Directions:

1. In a large skillet, heat the olive oil over medium heat. Add the onion and garlic and sauté until softened, about 5 minutes.
2. Add the ground turkey and cook until browned, breaking it up with a spoon, about 5-7 minutes.
3. Add the bell peppers, zucchini, and broccoli to the skillet. Cook for an additional 5-7 minutes, until the vegetables are tender-crisp.
4. Stir in the soy sauce, hoisin sauce, ginger, salt, and pepper. Cook for another 2-3 minutes, until everything is well combined and heated through.
5. Serve the stir-fry over cooked brown rice.

Serving: 4 servings

Nutrition (per serving):

Calories: 350
Protein: 28g
Fat: 18g
Carbohydrates: 20g
Fiber: 4g
Sugar: 6g

4. Quinoa and Black Bean Stuffed Peppers

Ingredients:

- 4 bell peppers, tops cut off and seeds removed
- 1 cup quinoa, rinsed
- 2 cups vegetable broth
- 1 can (15 oz) black beans, drained and rinsed
- 1 cup corn kernels
- 1 cup diced tomatoes
- 1 teaspoon cumin
- 1 teaspoon chili powder
- Salt and pepper to taste
- 1/2 cup shredded low-fat cheddar cheese (optional)
- Fresh cilantro, chopped (for garnish)

Directions:

1. Preheat the oven to 375°F (190°C).
2. In a medium saucepan, bring the vegetable broth to a boil. Add the quinoa, reduce heat, cover, and simmer for 15 minutes, or until the liquid is absorbed and the quinoa is tender. Fluff with a fork.

3. In a large bowl, combine the cooked quinoa, black beans, corn, diced tomatoes, cumin, chili powder, salt, and pepper.
4. Stuff the bell peppers with the quinoa mixture and place them in a baking dish.
5. Cover with foil and bake for 30 minutes. If using cheese, remove the foil, sprinkle cheese on top, and bake for an additional 5 minutes, or until the cheese is melted.
6. Garnish with fresh cilantro before serving.

Serving: 4 servings

Nutrition (per serving):

Calories: 290
Protein: 12g
Fat: 5g
Carbohydrates: 52g
Fiber: 12g
Sugar: 8g

5. Greek Yogurt Chicken Salad
Ingredients:

- 2 cups cooked chicken breast, chopped
- 1 cup plain Greek yogurt
- 1 tablespoon Dijon mustard
- 1/4 cup red onion, finely chopped
- 1/4 cup celery, finely chopped
- 1/4 cup apple, chopped
- 2 tablespoons fresh parsley, chopped
- 1 tablespoon fresh lemon juice
- Salt and pepper to taste
- Lettuce leaves (for serving)

Directions:

1. In a large bowl, combine the Greek yogurt, Dijon mustard, red onion, celery, apple, parsley, lemon juice, salt, and pepper.
2. Add the chopped chicken breast and stir until well combined.
3. Serve the chicken salad on lettuce leaves or as a sandwich filling.

Serving: 4 servings

Nutrition (per serving):

Calories: 200

Protein: 30g

Fat: 4g

Carbohydrates: 8g

Fiber: 1g

Sugar: 4g

Snack and Appetizer Recipes

8.1 Anti-inflammatory Snack Ideas

1. Almond Butter and Apple Slices
Ingredients:

- 1 apple, sliced
- 2 tablespoons almond butter

Directions:

1. Spread almond butter on apple slices.
2. Enjoy immediately.

Serving: 1 serving

Nutrition (per serving):

Calories: 210

Protein: 4g

Fat: 11g

Carbohydrates: 26g

Fiber: 7g

Sugar: 17g

2. Greek Yogurt with Berries
Ingredients:

- 1/2 cup Greek yogurt
- 1/2 cup mixed berries (blueberries, strawberries, raspberries)

- 1 tablespoon honey (optional)

Directions:

1. Place Greek yogurt in a bowl.
2. Top with mixed berries.
3. Drizzle with honey if desired.
4. Mix and enjoy.

Serving: 1 serving

Nutrition (per serving):

Calories: 150

Protein: 12g

Fat: 0g

Carbohydrates: 24g

Fiber: 3g

Sugar: 19g

3. Hummus and Veggie Sticks

Ingredients:

- 1/2 cup hummus
- Carrot sticks, cucumber slices, bell pepper strips (as desired)

Directions:

1. Place hummus in a small bowl.
2. Serve with veggie sticks.
3. Dip and enjoy.

Serving: 1 serving

Nutrition (per serving):

Calories: 180
Protein: 7g
Fat: 10g
Carbohydrates: 16g
Fiber: 6g
Sugar: 2g

4. Chia Seed Pudding

Ingredients:

- 1/4 cup chia seeds
- 1 cup unsweetened almond milk
- 1 tablespoon honey or maple syrup (optional)
- Fresh berries for topping

Directions:

1. In a bowl or jar, mix chia seeds and almond milk.
2. Add honey or maple syrup if desired.
3. Refrigerate for at least 2 hours or overnight, until mixture thickens.
4. Top with fresh berries before serving.

Serving: 1 serving

Nutrition (per serving):

Calories: 220
Protein: 6g
Fat: 12g
Carbohydrates: 24g

Fiber: 12g

Sugar: 8g

5. Avocado Toast

Ingredients:

- 1 slice whole grain bread, toasted
- 1/2 avocado, mashed
- Cherry tomatoes, sliced (optional)
- Sprinkle of sea salt and black pepper

Directions:

1. Spread mashed avocado on toasted bread.
2. Top with sliced cherry tomatoes if desired.
3. Season with sea salt and black pepper.
4. Enjoy immediately.

Serving: 1 serving

Nutrition (per serving):

Calories: 200

Protein: 5g

Fat: 11g

Carbohydrates: 23g

Fiber: 7g

Sugar: 2g

8.2 Quick and Healthy Appetizers

1. Caprese Skewers

Ingredients:

- Cherry tomatoes
- Fresh mozzarella balls (bocconcini)
- Fresh basil leaves
- Balsamic glaze
- Toothpicks

Directions:

1. Thread cherry tomatoes, mozzarella balls, and basil leaves onto toothpicks.
2. Arrange on a serving platter.
3. Drizzle with balsamic glaze.
4. Serve immediately.

Serving: Makes 12 skewers

Nutrition (per skewer):

Calories: 30

Protein: 2g

Fat: 2g

Carbohydrates: 2g

Fiber: 0g

Sugar: 1g

2. Guacamole with Veggie Chips

Ingredients:

- 2 ripe avocados
- 1/4 cup diced tomatoes
- 1/4 cup diced red onion
- 1 tablespoon lime juice
- Salt and pepper to taste
- Veggie chips (carrot, cucumber, bell pepper)

Directions:

1. In a bowl, mash avocados with a fork.
2. Stir in diced tomatoes, red onion, lime juice, salt, and pepper.
3. Serve with veggie chips.

Serving: Serves 4

Nutrition (per serving, including chips):

Calories: 160
Protein: 3g
Fat: 12g
Carbohydrates: 14g
Fiber: 8g
Sugar: 3g

3. Smoked Salmon Cucumber Bites

Ingredients:

- English cucumber, sliced into rounds
- Smoked salmon slices

- Cream cheese
- Fresh dill, for garnish

Directions:

1. Spread a thin layer of cream cheese on each cucumber slice.
2. Top with a piece of smoked salmon.
3. Garnish with fresh dill.
4. Arrange on a platter and serve.

Serving: Makes about 20 pieces

Nutrition (per piece):

Calories: 20
Protein: 2g
Fat: 1g
Carbohydrates: 1g
Fiber: 0g
Sugar: 0g

4. Stuffed Mini Bell Peppers

Ingredients:

- Mini bell peppers, halved and deseeded
- Hummus
- Cherry tomatoes, halved
- Fresh parsley, chopped

Directions:

1. Fill each mini bell pepper half with hummus.
2. Top with cherry tomato halves.

3. Garnish with chopped parsley.

4. Arrange on a platter and serve.

Serving: Makes about 16 pieces

Nutrition (per piece):

Calories: 15

Protein: 1g

Fat: 1g

Carbohydrates: 2g

Fiber: 1g

Sugar: 1g

5. Greek Yogurt Dip with Veggie Sticks

Ingredients:

- 1 cup plain Greek yogurt
- 1 tablespoon lemon juice
- 1 tablespoon chopped fresh dill
- 1/2 teaspoon garlic powder
- Salt and pepper to taste
- Assorted veggie sticks (carrot, celery, cucumber)

Directions:

1. In a bowl, mix Greek yogurt, lemon juice, dill, garlic powder, salt, and pepper.
2. Serve with assorted veggie sticks.

Serving: Serves 4

Nutrition (per serving, including veggie sticks):

Calories: 70

Protein: 8g

Fat: 0g

Carbohydrates: 10g

Fiber: 2g

Sugar: 6g

8.3 Nutrient-dense Snacks

1. Mixed Nuts and Dried Fruit

Ingredients:

- 1/4 cup mixed nuts (almonds, walnuts, cashews)
- 1/4 cup dried cranberries or apricots
- 1 tablespoon dark chocolate chips (optional)

Directions:

1. Combine mixed nuts, dried fruit, and dark chocolate chips (if using) in a small bowl.
2. Mix well.
3. Portion into individual servings or enjoy as a mix.

Serving: 1 serving

Nutrition (per serving):

Calories: 200
Protein: 5g
Fat: 12g
Carbohydrates: 20g
Fiber: 3g
Sugar: 12g

2. Cottage Cheese with Fresh Fruit

Ingredients:

- 1/2 cup low-fat cottage cheese
- 1/2 cup mixed fresh fruit (berries, pineapple, kiwi)

Directions:

1. Place cottage cheese in a bowl.
2. Top with mixed fresh fruit.
3. Serve immediately.

Serving: 1 serving

Nutrition (per serving):

Calories: 120
Protein: 14g
Fat: 2g
Carbohydrates: 14g
Fiber: 2g
Sugar: 10g

3. Edamame with Sea Salt

Ingredients:

- 1 cup edamame (frozen, thawed)
- Sea salt to taste

Directions:

1. Steam or microwave edamame until heated through.
2. Sprinkle with sea salt.
3. Enjoy warm or at room temperature.

Serving: 1 serving

Nutrition (per serving):

Calories: 120
Protein: 11g
Fat: 5g
Carbohydrates: 9g
Fiber: 5g
Sugar: 3g

4. Greek Yogurt with Chia Seeds and Honey

Ingredients:

- 1/2 cup plain Greek yogurt
- 1 tablespoon chia seeds
- 1 tablespoon honey

Directions:

1. In a bowl, combine Greek yogurt and chia seeds.
2. Drizzle with honey.
3. Mix well and enjoy.

Serving: 1 serving

Nutrition (per serving):

Calories: 180
Protein: 15g
Fat: 6g
Carbohydrates: 19g
Fiber: 3g
Sugar: 14g

5. Kale Chips

Ingredients:

- 1 bunch kale, washed and dried
- 1 tablespoon olive oil
- Sea salt to taste

Directions:

1. Preheat oven to 300°F (150°C).
2. Remove kale leaves from stems and tear into bite-sized pieces.
3. In a bowl, toss kale with olive oil and sea salt.
4. Spread kale in a single layer on a baking sheet.
5. Bake for 10-15 minutes, until crispy.
6. Let cool before serving.

Serving: Makes 2 servings

Nutrition (per serving):

Calories: 100

Protein: 5g

Fat: 7g

Carbohydrates: 10g

Fiber: 2g

Sugar: 1g

Dessert Recipes

9.1 Low-sugar and Anti-inflammatory Sweets

1. Chia Seed Pudding with Berries

Ingredients:

- 1/4 cup chia seeds
- 1 cup unsweetened almond milk
- 1 tablespoon honey or maple syrup (optional)
- Fresh berries for topping

Directions:

1. In a bowl or jar, mix chia seeds and almond milk.
2. Add honey or maple syrup if desired.
3. Refrigerate for at least 2 hours or overnight, until mixture thickens.
4. Top with fresh berries before serving.

Serving: 1 serving

Nutrition (per serving):

Calories: 220

Protein: 6g

Fat: 10g

Carbohydrates: 28g

Fiber: 12g

Sugar: 10g

2. Baked Apples with Cinnamon

Ingredients:

- 2 apples, cored
- 1 tablespoon melted coconut oil
- 1 teaspoon cinnamon
- 1 tablespoon chopped nuts (optional)

Directions:

1. Preheat oven to 375°F (190°C).
2. Place cored apples on a baking sheet.
3. Drizzle with melted coconut oil and sprinkle with cinnamon.
4. Bake for 20-25 minutes, until apples are tender.
5. Sprinkle with chopped nuts before serving.

Serving: 2 servings

Nutrition (per serving):

Calories: 150

Protein: 1g

Fat: 7g

Carbohydrates: 24g

Fiber: 5g

Sugar: 17g

3. Banana-Oat Cookies

Ingredients:

- 2 ripe bananas, mashed
- 1 cup rolled oats

- 1/4 cup chopped nuts (walnuts, almonds)
- 1/4 cup raisins or dried cranberries
- 1 teaspoon vanilla extract
- 1/2 teaspoon cinnamon

Directions:

1. Preheat oven to 350°F (175°C).
2. In a bowl, combine mashed bananas, rolled oats, chopped nuts, raisins or dried cranberries, vanilla extract, and cinnamon.
3. Drop spoonfuls of the mixture onto a baking sheet lined with parchment paper.
4. Flatten each cookie slightly with a fork.
5. Bake for 15-20 minutes, until golden brown.
6. Let cool before serving.

Serving: Makes about 12 cookies

Nutrition (per cookie):

Calories: 80
Protein: 2g
Fat: 3g
Carbohydrates: 13g
Fiber: 2g
Sugar: 5g

4. Coconut Mango Popsicles
Ingredients:

- 1 cup coconut milk
- 1 ripe mango, peeled and chopped
- 1 tablespoon honey or maple syrup (optional)

Directions:

1. In a blender, combine coconut milk, chopped mango, and honey or maple syrup if using.
2. Blend until smooth.
3. Pour mixture into popsicle molds.
4. Insert popsicle sticks and freeze for at least 4 hours, until solid.
5. Remove from molds and enjoy.

Serving: Makes 6 popsicles

Nutrition (per popsicle):

Calories: 90
Protein: 1g
Fat: 6g
Carbohydrates: 10g
Fiber: 1g
Sugar: 9g

5. Dark Chocolate Avocado Mousse

Ingredients:

- 2 ripe avocados
- 1/4 cup cocoa powder
- 1/4 cup honey or maple syrup
- 1 teaspoon vanilla extract
- Pinch of sea salt
- Fresh berries for topping

Directions:

1. In a blender or food processor, combine avocados, cocoa powder, honey or maple syrup, vanilla extract, and sea salt.
2. Blend until smooth and creamy.
3. Spoon into serving bowls.
4. Top with fresh berries before serving.

Serving: 4 servings

Nutrition (per serving):

Calories: 200

Protein: 3g

Fat: 12g

Carbohydrates: 26g

Fiber: 7g

Sugar: 15g

9.2 Healthy Baking Alternatives

1. Almond Flour Banana Bread

Ingredients:

- 2 ripe bananas, mashed
- 2 eggs
- 1/4 cup coconut oil, melted
- 1/4 cup honey or maple syrup
- 1 teaspoon vanilla extract
- 2 cups almond flour
- 1 teaspoon baking powder
- 1/2 teaspoon baking soda
- 1/2 teaspoon cinnamon
- Pinch of salt

Directions:

1. Preheat oven to 350°F (175°C). Grease or line a loaf pan with parchment paper.
2. In a bowl, mix mashed bananas, eggs, melted coconut oil, honey or maple syrup, and vanilla extract.
3. In another bowl, combine almond flour, baking powder, baking soda, cinnamon, and salt.
4. Gradually add dry ingredients to wet ingredients, stirring until well combined.
5. Pour batter into the prepared loaf pan.
6. Bake for 40-45 minutes, or until a toothpick inserted into the center comes out clean.
7. Allow to cool before slicing and serving.

Serving: Makes 10 slices

Nutrition (per slice):

Calories: 230

Protein: 6g

Fat: 16g

Carbohydrates: 18g

Fiber: 3g

Sugar: 10g

2. Oatmeal Raisin Cookies

Ingredients:

- 1 cup rolled oats
- 1/2 cup almond flour
- 1/2 teaspoon baking soda
- 1/2 teaspoon cinnamon
- Pinch of salt
- 1/4 cup coconut oil, melted
- 1/4 cup honey or maple syrup
- 1 egg
- 1 teaspoon vanilla extract
- 1/2 cup raisins

Directions:

1. Preheat oven to 350°F (175°C). Line a baking sheet with parchment paper.
2. In a bowl, combine rolled oats, almond flour, baking soda, cinnamon, and salt.
3. In another bowl, whisk together melted coconut oil, honey or maple syrup, egg, and vanilla extract.
4. Gradually add dry ingredients to wet ingredients, stirring until well combined.
5. Fold in raisins.

6. Drop spoonfuls of dough onto the prepared baking sheet.

7. Flatten each cookie slightly with a fork.

8. Bake for 12-15 minutes, or until edges are golden brown.

9. Allow to cool before serving.

Serving: Makes about 12 cookies

Nutrition (per cookie):

Calories: 140

Protein: 3g

Fat: 7g

Carbohydrates: 18g

Fiber: 2g

Sugar: 8g

3. Sweet Potato Brownies

Ingredients:

- 1 cup cooked and mashed sweet potato
- 1/4 cup almond butter
- 1/4 cup honey or maple syrup
- 1 egg
- 1 teaspoon vanilla extract
- 1/4 cup cocoa powder
- 1/2 teaspoon baking soda
- Pinch of salt
- 1/4 cup dark chocolate chips (optional)

Directions:

1. Preheat oven to 350°F (175°C). Grease or line a baking dish with parchment paper.
2. In a bowl, mix mashed sweet potato, almond butter, honey or maple syrup, egg, and vanilla extract until smooth.
3. Add cocoa powder, baking soda, and salt, stirring until well combined.
4. Fold in dark chocolate chips if using.
5. Pour batter into the prepared baking dish, spreading evenly.
6. Bake for 20-25 minutes, or until a toothpick inserted into the center comes out clean.
7. Allow to cool before cutting into squares and serving.

Serving: Makes 9 brownies

Nutrition (per brownie):

Calories: 150
Protein: 4g
Fat: 8g
Carbohydrates: 18g
Fiber: 2g
Sugar: 10g

4. Coconut Flour Pancakes

Ingredients:

- 1/4 cup coconut flour
- 1/2 teaspoon baking powder
- Pinch of salt
- 2 eggs
- 1/4 cup coconut milk
- 1 tablespoon honey or maple syrup

- 1/2 teaspoon vanilla extract
- Coconut oil or butter for cooking

Directions:

1. In a bowl, whisk together coconut flour, baking powder, and salt.
2. In another bowl, whisk eggs, coconut milk, honey or maple syrup, and vanilla extract.
3. Gradually add dry ingredients to wet ingredients, stirring until well combined.
4. Heat coconut oil or butter in a skillet over medium heat.
5. Pour batter onto the skillet to form pancakes (about 2-3 tablespoons per pancake).
6. Cook for 2-3 minutes on each side, until golden brown.
7. Repeat with remaining batter.
8. Serve warm with toppings of your choice.

Serving: Makes 6 small pancakes

Nutrition (per pancake, without toppings):

Calories: 70

Protein: 3g

Fat: 4g

Carbohydrates: 6g

Fiber: 2g

Sugar: 3g

5. Lemon Poppy Seed Muffins
Ingredients:

- 1 cup almond flour
- 1/4 cup coconut flour

- 1/4 cup honey or maple syrup
- 1/4 cup melted coconut oil
- 3 eggs
- Juice and zest of 1 lemon
- 1 tablespoon poppy seeds
- 1/2 teaspoon baking soda
- Pinch of salt

Directions:

1. Preheat oven to 350°F (175°C). Line a muffin tin with paper liners.
2. In a bowl, whisk together almond flour, coconut flour, honey or maple syrup, melted coconut oil, eggs, lemon juice and zest, poppy seeds, baking soda, and salt until smooth.
3. Divide batter evenly among muffin cups.
4. Bake for 18-20 minutes, or until a toothpick inserted into the center comes out clean.
5. Allow to cool before serving.

Serving: Makes 8 muffins

Nutrition (per muffin):

Calories: 200
Protein: 5g
Fat: 14g
Carbohydrates: 15g
Fiber: 3g
Sugar: 9g

9.3 Fruit-based Desserts

1. Mixed Fruit Salad

Ingredients:

- 1 cup strawberries, sliced
- 1 cup pineapple chunks
- 1 cup grapes, halved
- 1 banana, sliced
- Fresh mint leaves for garnish

Directions:

1. Combine all fruits in a bowl.
2. Toss gently to mix.
3. Garnish with fresh mint leaves.
4. Serve immediately or chill before serving.

Serving: Makes 4 servings

Nutrition (per serving):

Calories: 100
Protein: 1g
Fat: 0.5g
Carbohydrates: 25g
Fiber: 3g
Sugar: 18g

2. Mango Coconut Chia Pudding

Ingredients:

- 1/2 cup chia seeds
- 1 1/2 cups unsweetened coconut milk
- 1 ripe mango, diced
- 1 tablespoon honey or maple syrup (optional)

Directions:

1. In a bowl, mix chia seeds and coconut milk.
2. Stir in diced mango and sweetener if using.
3. Refrigerate for at least 2 hours or overnight until thickened.
4. Serve chilled.

Serving: Makes 2 servings

Nutrition (per serving):

Calories: 300
Protein: 7g
Fat: 15g
Carbohydrates: 40g
Fiber: 15g
Sugar: 20g

3. Berry Frozen Yogurt Bites

Ingredients:

- 1 cup mixed berries (blueberries, raspberries, strawberries)
- 1 cup Greek yogurt
- 1 tablespoon honey (optional)

Directions:

1. Line a mini muffin tin with paper liners.
2. In a bowl, mix Greek yogurt and honey.
3. Spoon a layer of yogurt into each muffin cup.
4. Add a few berries on top.
5. Repeat layers until cups are filled.
6. Freeze for 2-3 hours until firm.
7. Remove from muffin tin and serve.

Serving: Makes 12 bites

Nutrition (per bite):

Calories: 30

Protein: 2g

Fat: 0g

Carbohydrates: 5g

Fiber: 1g

Sugar: 4g

4. Grilled Pineapple with Honey and Cinnamon

Ingredients:

- 1 pineapple, peeled and sliced into rings
- 2 tablespoons honey
- 1/2 teaspoon ground cinnamon

Directions:

1. Preheat grill or grill pan over medium-high heat.
2. Grill pineapple slices for 2-3 minutes per side until grill marks appear.

3. Remove from heat and drizzle with honey.
4. Sprinkle with ground cinnamon.
5. Serve warm.

Serving: Makes 4 servings

Nutrition (per serving):

Calories: 120
Protein: 1g
Fat: 0g
Carbohydrates: 32g
Fiber: 3g
Sugar: 25g

5. Fruit and Yogurt Popsicles

Ingredients:

- 1 cup mixed berries (strawberries, blueberries, raspberries)
- 1 cup Greek yogurt
- 1 tablespoon honey or maple syrup (optional)

Directions:

1. In a blender, puree mixed berries with honey or maple syrup.
2. Fill popsicle molds halfway with berry puree.
3. Top with Greek yogurt.
4. Insert popsicle sticks and freeze for 4-6 hours until solid.
5. Remove from molds and serve.

Serving: Makes 6 popsicles

Nutrition (per popsicle):

Calories: 70
Protein: 4g
Fat: 0.5g
Carbohydrates: 14g
Fiber: 2g
Sugar: 10g

Beverage Recipes

10.1 Anti-inflammatory Teas and Tonics

1. Turmeric Ginger Tea
Ingredients:

- 1 cup water
- 1 teaspoon grated fresh turmeric (or 1/2 teaspoon ground turmeric)
- 1 teaspoon grated fresh ginger
- 1 teaspoon honey (optional)
- Juice of half a lemon

Directions:

1. In a small saucepan, bring water to a boil.
2. Add grated turmeric and ginger.
3. Reduce heat and simmer for 5-7 minutes.
4. Strain into a mug.
5. Stir in honey and lemon juice.
6. Enjoy warm.

Serving: 1 serving

Nutrition (per serving, without honey):

Calories: 5
Protein: 0g
Fat: 0g
Carbohydrates: 1g
Fiber: 0g

Sugar: 0g

2. Green Tea with Lemon and Mint

Ingredients:

- 1 cup water
- 1 green tea bag
- Juice of half a lemon
- Fresh mint leaves

Directions:

1. Bring water to a boil.
2. Steep green tea bag in hot water for 3-5 minutes.
3. Remove tea bag and pour tea into a mug.
4. Stir in lemon juice.
5. Garnish with fresh mint leaves.
6. Enjoy hot or chilled.

Serving: 1 serving

Nutrition (per serving):

Calories: 0

Protein: 0g

Fat: 0g

Carbohydrates: 0g

Fiber: 0g

Sugar: 0g

3. Hibiscus Ginger Iced Tea

Ingredients:

- 2 cups water
- 2 tablespoons dried hibiscus flowers
- 1 teaspoon grated fresh ginger
- 1 tablespoon honey (optional)
- Ice cubes
- Fresh lemon slices (optional)

Directions:

1. In a saucepan, bring water to a boil.
2. Add hibiscus flowers and grated ginger.
3. Remove from heat and let steep for 10-15 minutes.
4. Strain into a pitcher.
5. Stir in honey while tea is still warm.
6. Refrigerate until chilled.
7. Serve over ice with fresh lemon slices if desired.

Serving: Makes 2 servings

Nutrition (per serving, without honey):

Calories: 5

Protein: 0g

Fat: 0g

Carbohydrates: 1g

Fiber: 0g

Sugar: 0g

4. Chamomile Lavender Sleep Tonic

Ingredients:

- 1 cup water
- 1 chamomile tea bag
- 1 teaspoon dried lavender flowers
- 1 teaspoon honey (optional)

Directions:

1. Bring water to a boil.
2. Steep chamomile tea bag and dried lavender flowers in hot water for 5-7 minutes.
3. Remove tea bag and strain tonic into a mug.
4. Stir in honey if desired.
5. Enjoy warm before bedtime.

Serving: 1 serving

Nutrition (per serving, without honey):

Calories: 0
Protein: 0g
Fat: 0g
Carbohydrates: 0g
Fiber: 0g
Sugar: 0g

5. Golden Milk Turmeric Latte

Ingredients:

- 1 cup unsweetened almond milk (or any milk of choice)
- 1/2 teaspoon ground turmeric

- 1/4 teaspoon ground cinnamon
- Pinch of ground black pepper
- 1 teaspoon honey or maple syrup (optional)
- 1/2 teaspoon grated fresh ginger (optional)

Directions:

1. In a small saucepan, heat almond milk over medium heat.
2. Whisk in turmeric, cinnamon, black pepper, and grated ginger if using.
3. Heat until warm but not boiling, whisking occasionally.
4. Remove from heat and stir in honey or maple syrup if desired.
5. Pour into a mug and enjoy warm.

Serving: 1 serving

Nutrition (per serving, without honey):

Calories: 40
Protein: 1g
Fat: 3g
Carbohydrates: 3g
Fiber: 1g
Sugar: 1g

10.2 Smoothies and Juices

1. Berry Blast Smoothie

Ingredients:

- 1 cup mixed berries (strawberries, blueberries, raspberries)
- 1 banana
- 1/2 cup Greek yogurt
- 1 tablespoon honey or maple syrup
- 1/2 cup almond milk (or any milk of choice)
- Ice cubes (optional)

Directions:

1. Add all ingredients to a blender.
2. Blend until smooth.
3. If desired, add ice cubes and blend again until desired consistency is reached.
4. Pour into a glass and serve immediately.

Serving: Makes 2 servings

Nutrition (per serving):

Calories: 200
Protein: 8g
Fat: 3g
Carbohydrates: 40g
Fiber: 6g
Sugar: 28g

2. Green Goddess Smoothie

Ingredients:

- 1 cup spinach leaves
- 1/2 cup cucumber, chopped
- 1/2 avocado
- 1/2 cup pineapple chunks
- Juice of half a lemon
- 1 cup coconut water (or water)

Directions:

1. Place spinach, cucumber, avocado, pineapple, and lemon juice in a blender.
2. Add coconut water (or water).
3. Blend until smooth.
4. Pour into glasses and serve immediately.

Serving: Makes 1-2 servings

Nutrition (per serving):

Calories: 180
Protein: 4g
Fat: 9g
Carbohydrates: 24g
Fiber: 9g
Sugar: 11g

3. Tropical Turmeric Smoothie

Ingredients:

- 1 cup mango chunks

- 1 banana
- 1/2 teaspoon ground turmeric
- 1/2 teaspoon grated fresh ginger
- 1 tablespoon chia seeds
- 1 cup coconut water (or water)

Directions:

1. Add mango, banana, turmeric, ginger, chia seeds, and coconut water to a blender.
2. Blend until smooth.
3. Pour into glasses and serve immediately.

Serving: Makes 1-2 servings

Nutrition (per serving):

Calories: 230
Protein: 5g
Fat: 4g
Carbohydrates: 48g
Fiber: 9g
Sugar: 32g

4. Carrot Ginger Citrus Juice

Ingredients:

- 4 large carrots, peeled and chopped
- 1 orange, peeled and segmented
- 1/2 inch piece of fresh ginger
- Juice of half a lemon
- 1 cup water

Directions:

1. Place carrots, orange segments, ginger, lemon juice, and water in a blender.
2. Blend until smooth.
3. Strain through a fine mesh sieve or nut milk bag to extract juice.
4. Serve chilled over ice if desired.

Serving: Makes 2 servings

Nutrition (per serving):

Calories: 100
Protein: 2g
Fat: 0g
Carbohydrates: 24g
Fiber: 6g
Sugar: 14g

5. Pineapple Mint Green Juice

Ingredients:

- 2 cups fresh pineapple chunks
- 1 cucumber, peeled and chopped
- 1 cup spinach leaves
- Juice of 1 lime
- Handful of fresh mint leaves
- 1 cup coconut water (or water)

Directions:

1. Place pineapple, cucumber, spinach, lime juice, mint leaves, and coconut water in a blender.

2. Blend until smooth.

3. Strain through a fine mesh sieve or nut milk bag to extract juice.

4. Serve chilled over ice if desired.

Serving: Makes 2 servings

Nutrition (per serving):

Calories: 130

Protein: 3g

Fat: 1g

Carbohydrates: 32g

Fiber: 5g

Sugar: 20g

10.3 Hydrating and Healing Drinks

1. Cucumber Mint Infused Water

Ingredients:

- 1 cucumber, sliced
- Handful of fresh mint leaves
- 4 cups water
- Ice cubes (optional)

Directions:

1. In a pitcher, combine cucumber slices and fresh mint leaves.
2. Add water.
3. Refrigerate for at least 1 hour to allow flavors to infuse.
4. Serve over ice if desired.

Serving: Makes 4 servings

Nutrition (per serving):

Calories: 0
Protein: 0g
Fat: 0g
Carbohydrates: 0g
Fiber: 0g
Sugar: 0g

2. Ginger Lemonade

Ingredients:

- 4 cups water

- Juice of 4 lemons
- 1/4 cup honey or maple syrup
- 1 tablespoon grated fresh ginger
- Ice cubes
- Lemon slices for garnish

Directions:

1. In a pitcher, combine water, lemon juice, honey or maple syrup, and grated ginger.
2. Stir until honey or maple syrup is dissolved.
3. Refrigerate for at least 30 minutes.
4. Serve over ice with lemon slices for garnish.

Serving: Makes 4 servings

Nutrition (per serving):

Calories: 70
Protein: 0g
Fat: 0g
Carbohydrates: 19g
Fiber: 0g
Sugar: 16g

3. Coconut Water Electrolyte Drink

Ingredients:

- 2 cups coconut water
- Juice of 1 lime
- 1/4 teaspoon sea salt
- 1 tablespoon honey or maple syrup (optional)

Directions:

1. In a glass, combine coconut water, lime juice, sea salt, and honey or maple syrup if using.
2. Stir until well combined.
3. Serve chilled or over ice.

Serving: Makes 2 servings

Nutrition (per serving, without honey):

Calories: 45
Protein: 1g
Fat: 0g
Carbohydrates: 11g
Fiber: 0g
Sugar: 9g

4. Aloe Vera Limeade

Ingredients:

- 1/2 cup fresh aloe vera gel (scoop out the gel from the leaf)
- 3 cups water
- Juice of 2 limes
- 2 tablespoons honey or maple syrup
- Ice cubes

Directions:

1. In a blender, combine aloe vera gel, water, lime juice, and honey or maple syrup.
2. Blend until smooth.
3. Pour over ice cubes in glasses.

4. Serve immediately.

Serving: Makes 2 servings

Nutrition (per serving):

Calories: 80

Protein: 0g

Fat: 0g

Carbohydrates: 22g

Fiber: 0g

Sugar: 18g

5. Chamomile Lavender Tea

Ingredients:

- 2 cups water
- 2 chamomile tea bags
- 1 teaspoon dried lavender flowers
- Honey or maple syrup to taste (optional)

Directions:

1. Bring water to a boil in a saucepan.
2. Remove from heat and add chamomile tea bags and dried lavender flowers.
3. Cover and steep for 5-10 minutes.
4. Strain into mugs and sweeten with honey or maple syrup if desired.
5. Serve warm.

Serving: Makes 2 servings

Nutrition (per serving, without sweetener):

Calories: 0
Protein: 0g
Fat: 0g
Carbohydrates: 0g
Fiber: 0g
Sugar: 0g

Special Diets and Modifications

11.1 Gluten-free Recipes

1 Gluten-free Quinoa Salad

Ingredients:

- 1 cup quinoa, rinsed
- 2 cups water or vegetable broth
- 1/2 cup cherry tomatoes, halved
- 1/2 cucumber, diced
- 1/4 cup red onion, finely chopped
- 1/4 cup fresh parsley, chopped
- 1/4 cup feta cheese, crumbled (optional)
- Juice of 1 lemon
- 2 tablespoons olive oil
- Salt and pepper to taste

Directions:

1. In a medium saucepan, bring water or vegetable broth to a boil.
2. Add quinoa, reduce heat to low, cover, and simmer for 15 minutes or until quinoa is cooked and liquid is absorbed.
3. Fluff quinoa with a fork and let it cool to room temperature.
4. In a large bowl, combine cooked quinoa, cherry tomatoes, cucumber, red onion, parsley, and feta cheese.
5. In a small bowl, whisk together lemon juice, olive oil, salt, and pepper.
6. Pour dressing over quinoa salad and toss gently to combine.
7. Serve chilled or at room temperature.

Serving: Makes 4 servings

Nutrition (per serving):

Calories: 250
Protein: 8g
Fat: 10g
Carbohydrates: 33g
Fiber: 4g
Sugar: 2g

2 Gluten-free Chicken Stir Fry
Ingredients:

- 1 lb boneless, skinless chicken breasts, sliced thinly
- 2 tablespoons gluten-free soy sauce or tamari
- 1 tablespoon cornstarch
- 2 tablespoons olive oil
- 1 bell pepper, sliced
- 1 cup broccoli florets
- 1 carrot, sliced
- 2 cloves garlic, minced
- 1 tablespoon grated fresh ginger
- Salt and pepper to taste
- Cooked rice or quinoa for serving

Directions:

1. In a bowl, toss sliced chicken with gluten-free soy sauce and cornstarch until well coated.
2. Heat olive oil in a large skillet or wok over medium-high heat.

3. Add chicken and cook until browned and cooked through, about 5-7 minutes. Remove from skillet and set aside.
4. In the same skillet, add bell pepper, broccoli, carrot, garlic, and ginger. Stir-fry for 3-4 minutes until vegetables are tender-crisp.
5. Return chicken to the skillet and toss to combine with vegetables.
6. Season with salt and pepper to taste.
7. Serve hot over cooked rice or quinoa.

Serving: Makes 4 servings

Nutrition (per serving, without rice or quinoa):

Calories: 280
Protein: 25g
Fat: 12g
Carbohydrates: 15g
Fiber: 3g
Sugar: 5g

3 Gluten-free Cauliflower Pizza Crust

Ingredients:

- 1 medium head cauliflower, grated (about 4 cups)
- 1/2 cup grated Parmesan cheese
- 1 teaspoon dried oregano
- 1/2 teaspoon garlic powder
- 1/4 teaspoon salt
- 1 egg, beaten
- 1/4 cup almond flour or gluten-free flour blend
- Pizza sauce, cheese, and toppings of choice

Directions:

1. Preheat oven to 400°F (200°C). Line a baking sheet with parchment paper.
2. Place grated cauliflower in a microwave-safe bowl and microwave on high for 5-6 minutes until softened.
3. Let cauliflower cool slightly, then transfer to a clean kitchen towel or cheesecloth. Squeeze out excess moisture.
4. In a large bowl, combine cauliflower, Parmesan cheese, oregano, garlic powder, salt, egg, and almond flour or gluten-free flour blend. Mix until well combined.
5. Press cauliflower mixture onto the prepared baking sheet, forming a thin crust.
6. Bake for 20-25 minutes until crust is golden brown and edges are crispy.
7. Remove from oven and top with pizza sauce, cheese, and toppings of choice.
8. Return to oven and bake for an additional 10-15 minutes until cheese is melted and bubbly.
9. Slice and serve hot.

Serving: Makes 4 servings (1 small pizza crust)

Nutrition (per serving, crust only):

Calories: 120
Protein: 8g
Fat: 7g
Carbohydrates: 10g
Fiber: 4g
Sugar: 3g

4 Gluten-free Lentil Soup
Ingredients:

- 1 cup dried green lentils, rinsed

- 4 cups vegetable broth
- 1 onion, diced
- 2 carrots, diced
- 2 celery stalks, diced
- 2 cloves garlic, minced
- 1 teaspoon dried thyme
- 1 teaspoon ground cumin
- Salt and pepper to taste
- Fresh parsley for garnish

Directions:

1. In a large pot, combine lentils, vegetable broth, onion, carrots, celery, garlic, thyme, and cumin.
2. Bring to a boil, then reduce heat to low and simmer for 25-30 minutes until lentils and vegetables are tender.
3. Season with salt and pepper to taste.
4. Serve hot, garnished with fresh parsley if desired.

Serving: Makes 4 servings

Nutrition (per serving):

Calories: 250
Protein: 15g
Fat: 1g
Carbohydrates: 45g
Fiber: 15g
Sugar: 6g

5 Gluten-free Banana Oat Pancakes

Ingredients:

- 2 ripe bananas
- 2 eggs
- 1/2 cup rolled oats (certified gluten-free)
- 1/2 teaspoon baking powder
- 1/2 teaspoon ground cinnamon
- Coconut oil or butter for cooking
- Maple syrup and fresh fruit for serving

Directions:

1. In a blender, combine bananas, eggs, rolled oats, baking powder, and cinnamon. Blend until smooth.
2. Heat coconut oil or butter in a non-stick skillet over medium heat.
3. Pour batter onto the skillet to form pancakes (about 1/4 cup batter per pancake).
4. Cook for 2-3 minutes until bubbles form on the surface. Flip and cook for an additional 1-2 minutes until golden brown.
5. Repeat with remaining batter.
6. Serve warm with maple syrup and fresh fruit.

Serving: Makes 8 pancakes (2-4 servings)

Nutrition (per serving, 2 pancakes):

Calories: 250
Protein: 8g
Fat: 8g
Carbohydrates: 38g
Fiber: 5g
Sugar: 15g

11.2 Dairy-free Recipes

1 Dairy-free Coconut Curry Lentil Soup

Ingredients:

- 1 cup dried lentils, rinsed
- 4 cups vegetable broth
- 1 onion, diced
- 2 cloves garlic, minced
- 1 tablespoon grated ginger
- 1 red bell pepper, diced
- 1 carrot, diced
- 1 can (14 oz) coconut milk
- 2 tablespoons curry powder
- 1 teaspoon turmeric powder
- 1 tablespoon olive oil
- Salt and pepper to taste
- Fresh cilantro for garnish (optional)

Directions:

1. In a large pot, heat olive oil over medium heat. Add diced onion, garlic, and grated ginger. Sauté until onions are translucent.
2. Add diced bell pepper and carrot to the pot. Cook for 5-7 minutes until vegetables are slightly softened.
3. Stir in curry powder and turmeric powder, cook for 1 minute until fragrant.
4. Add rinsed lentils and vegetable broth to the pot. Bring to a boil, then reduce heat to low and simmer for 20-25 minutes until lentils are tender.
5. Stir in coconut milk and simmer for another 5 minutes to heat through.
6. Season with salt and pepper to taste.
7. Serve hot, garnished with fresh cilantro if desired.

Serving: Makes 4 servings

Nutrition (per serving):

Calories: 380

Protein: 14g

Fat: 21g

Carbohydrates: 36g

Fiber: 15g

Sugar: 4g

2 Dairy-free Chickpea Coconut Curry

Ingredients:

- 1 tablespoon coconut oil
- 1 onion, diced
- 2 cloves garlic, minced
- 1 tablespoon grated ginger
- 1 red bell pepper, diced
- 1 can (14 oz) chickpeas, drained and rinsed
- 1 can (14 oz) coconut milk
- 1 cup vegetable broth
- 2 tablespoons curry powder
- 1 teaspoon turmeric powder
- Salt and pepper to taste
- Fresh cilantro for garnish (optional)

Directions:

1. In a large skillet or pot, heat coconut oil over medium heat. Add diced onion, garlic, and grated ginger. Sauté until onions are translucent.

2. Add diced bell pepper to the skillet. Cook for 3-4 minutes until slightly softened.

3. Stir in curry powder and turmeric powder, cook for 1 minute until fragrant.

4. Add chickpeas, coconut milk, and vegetable broth to the skillet. Bring to a simmer and cook for 15-20 minutes, stirring occasionally, until the sauce thickens slightly.

5. Season with salt and pepper to taste.

6. Serve hot, garnished with fresh cilantro if desired, over rice or quinoa.

Serving: Makes 4 servings

Nutrition (per serving):

Calories: 380

Protein: 12g

Fat: 22g

Carbohydrates: 38g

Fiber: 9g

Sugar: 6g

3 Dairy-free Avocado Chocolate Mousse

Ingredients:

- 2 ripe avocados, peeled and pitted
- 1/4 cup cocoa powder
- 1/4 cup maple syrup or agave nectar
- 1 teaspoon vanilla extract
- Pinch of salt
- Fresh berries for garnish (optional)

Directions:

1. In a food processor or blender, combine avocado flesh, cocoa powder, maple syrup or agave nectar, vanilla extract, and salt.
2. Blend until smooth and creamy, scraping down the sides as needed.
3. Transfer mousse to serving bowls or glasses.
4. Refrigerate for at least 30 minutes to chill.
5. Serve cold, garnished with fresh berries if desired.

Serving: Makes 4 servings

Nutrition (per serving):

Calories: 200
Protein: 3g
Fat: 13g
Carbohydrates: 24g
Fiber: 7g
Sugar: 13g

4 Dairy-free Coconut Chia Pudding
Ingredients:

- 1/4 cup chia seeds
- 1 cup coconut milk
- 1 tablespoon maple syrup or agave nectar
- 1/2 teaspoon vanilla extract
- Fresh fruit for topping (such as berries or mango)

Directions:

1. In a bowl, whisk together chia seeds, coconut milk, maple syrup or agave nectar, and vanilla extract.
2. Cover and refrigerate for at least 2 hours or overnight, stirring occasionally, until mixture thickens into a pudding-like consistency.
3. Serve chilled, topped with fresh fruit.

Serving: Makes 2 servings

Nutrition (per serving):

Calories: 250

Protein: 5g

Fat: 20g

Carbohydrates: 16g

Fiber: 10g

Sugar: 5g

5 Dairy-free Banana Oatmeal Breakfast Cookies

Ingredients:

- 2 ripe bananas, mashed
- 1/4 cup coconut oil, melted
- 1/4 cup maple syrup or agave nectar
- 1 teaspoon vanilla extract
- 2 cups rolled oats (certified gluten-free if needed)
- 1/2 cup shredded coconut
- 1/2 cup raisins or chocolate chips (optional)
- 1 teaspoon cinnamon
- 1/2 teaspoon baking powder

- Pinch of salt

Directions:

1. Preheat oven to 350°F (175°C). Line a baking sheet with parchment paper.
2. In a large bowl, combine mashed bananas, melted coconut oil, maple syrup or agave nectar, and vanilla extract.
3. Add rolled oats, shredded coconut, raisins or chocolate chips if using, cinnamon, baking powder, and salt. Mix until well combined.
4. Drop spoonfuls of cookie dough onto the prepared baking sheet, spacing them apart.
5. Flatten each cookie slightly with the back of a spoon.
6. Bake for 15-18 minutes until edges are golden brown.
7. Remove from oven and let cool on the baking sheet for 5 minutes before transferring to a wire rack to cool completely.

Serving: Makes about 12 cookies

Nutrition (per cookie):

Calories: 180
Protein: 3g
Fat: 9g
Carbohydrates: 24g
Fiber: 3g
Sugar: 10g

11.3 Vegetarian and Vegan Options

1 Chickpea Spinach Curry

Ingredients:

- 1 tablespoon coconut oil
- 1 onion, finely chopped
- 2 cloves garlic, minced
- 1 tablespoon grated ginger
- 1 teaspoon ground cumin
- 1 teaspoon ground coriander
- 1/2 teaspoon turmeric powder
- 1/2 teaspoon paprika
- 1/4 teaspoon cayenne pepper (optional, for heat)
- 1 can (14 oz) diced tomatoes
- 1 can (14 oz) coconut milk
- 2 cups cooked chickpeas (or 1 can, drained and rinsed)
- 4 cups fresh spinach leaves
- Juice of 1/2 lemon
- Salt and pepper to taste
- Fresh cilantro for garnish (optional)

Directions:

1. In a large skillet or pot, heat coconut oil over medium heat. Add chopped onion and sauté until softened, about 5 minutes.
2. Add minced garlic and grated ginger, cook for 1-2 minutes until fragrant.
3. Stir in ground cumin, ground coriander, turmeric powder, paprika, and cayenne pepper (if using). Cook for another minute.
4. Add diced tomatoes (with juices) and coconut milk to the skillet. Bring to a simmer and cook for 10 minutes, stirring occasionally.

5. Add cooked chickpeas to the skillet and cook for 5 minutes to heat through.

6. Stir in fresh spinach leaves and cook until wilted, about 2-3 minutes.

7. Remove from heat and stir in lemon juice. Season with salt and pepper to taste.

8. Serve hot, garnished with fresh cilantro if desired, and with rice or naan bread.

Serving: Makes 4 servings

Nutrition (per serving, curry only):

Calories: 320

Protein: 11g

Fat: 18g

Carbohydrates: 32g

Fiber: 9g

Sugar: 6g

2 Vegan Quinoa Salad with Roasted Vegetables

Ingredients:

- 1 cup quinoa
- 2 cups vegetable broth
- 1 red bell pepper, diced
- 1 zucchini, diced
- 1 eggplant, diced
- 1 red onion, diced
- 2 tablespoons olive oil
- Salt and pepper to taste
- 1 cup cherry tomatoes, halved
- 1/4 cup chopped fresh parsley
- Juice of 1 lemon

Directions:

1. Preheat oven to 400°F (200°C). Line a baking sheet with parchment paper.
2. Toss diced red bell pepper, zucchini, eggplant, and red onion with olive oil, salt, and pepper. Spread on the prepared baking sheet.
3. Roast vegetables in the preheated oven for 25-30 minutes, until tender and slightly caramelized.
4. Meanwhile, rinse quinoa under cold water. In a medium saucepan, bring vegetable broth to a boil. Add quinoa, reduce heat to low, cover, and simmer for 15 minutes until quinoa is cooked and liquid is absorbed. Fluff with a fork.
5. In a large bowl, combine cooked quinoa, roasted vegetables, cherry tomatoes, chopped parsley, and lemon juice. Toss to mix well.
6. Serve warm or chilled.

Serving: Makes 4 servings

Nutrition (per serving):

Calories: 250
Protein: 7g
Fat: 10g
Carbohydrates: 35g
Fiber: 6g
Sugar: 7g

3 Vegan Lentil Shepherd's Pie
Ingredients:

- 1 cup green or brown lentils, rinsed
- 2 cups vegetable broth
- 1 onion, diced

- 2 cloves garlic, minced
- 2 carrots, diced
- 1 cup frozen peas
- 1 cup corn kernels
- 2 tablespoons tomato paste
- 1 teaspoon dried thyme
- Salt and pepper to taste
- 4 cups mashed potatoes (prepared with vegan butter and plant-based milk)

Directions:

1. Preheat oven to 375°F (190°C).
2. In a medium pot, combine lentils and vegetable broth. Bring to a boil, then reduce heat and simmer for 25-30 minutes until lentils are tender.
3. In a large skillet, sauté diced onion and minced garlic until softened. Add diced carrots and cook for another 5 minutes.
4. Stir in cooked lentils, peas, corn, tomato paste, dried thyme, salt, and pepper. Cook for 5-7 minutes until heated through.
5. Transfer lentil mixture to a baking dish and spread mashed potatoes evenly over the top.
6. Bake in the preheated oven for 20-25 minutes until the top is lightly browned.
7. Let cool slightly before serving.

Serving: Makes 6 servings

Nutrition (per serving):

Calories: 300
Protein: 10g
Fat: 5g
Carbohydrates: 54g
Fiber: 12g

Sugar: 6g

4 Vegan Sweet Potato and Black Bean Tacos
Ingredients:

- 2 medium sweet potatoes, peeled and diced
- 1 tablespoon olive oil
- 1 teaspoon cumin
- 1 teaspoon smoked paprika
- 1/2 teaspoon chili powder
- Salt and pepper to taste
- 1 can (14 oz) black beans, drained and rinsed
- 8 small corn tortillas
- 1 avocado, sliced
- Fresh cilantro for garnish
- Lime wedges for serving

Directions:

1. Preheat oven to 400°F (200°C). Line a baking sheet with parchment paper.
2. Toss diced sweet potatoes with olive oil, cumin, smoked paprika, chili powder, salt, and pepper. Spread on the prepared baking sheet.
3. Roast in the preheated oven for 25-30 minutes until tender and slightly caramelized.
4. Warm corn tortillas in a dry skillet over medium heat or in the oven.
5. Fill each tortilla with roasted sweet potatoes, black beans, avocado slices, and fresh cilantro.
6. Serve with lime wedges for squeezing over the tacos.

Serving: Makes 4 servings (2 tacos each)

Nutrition (per serving):

Calories: 350

Protein: 10g

Fat: 14g

Carbohydrates: 50g

Fiber: 14g

Sugar: 7g

5 Vegan Mushroom Stroganoff

Ingredients:

- 1 tablespoon olive oil
- 1 onion, diced
- 2 cloves garlic, minced
- 1 pound mushrooms, sliced
- 1 teaspoon dried thyme
- 1 teaspoon paprika
- 2 tablespoons flour (or gluten-free flour)
- 1 cup vegetable broth
- 1 cup unsweetened almond milk
- 2 tablespoons nutritional yeast
- 2 tablespoons soy sauce (or tamari for gluten-free)
- Salt and pepper to taste
- 8 oz whole wheat or gluten-free pasta

Directions:

1. Cook pasta according to package instructions. Drain and set aside.
2. In a large skillet, heat olive oil over medium heat. Add diced onion and sauté until softened, about 5 minutes.

3. Add minced garlic and cook for 1 minute until fragrant.

4. Stir in sliced mushrooms, dried thyme, and paprika. Cook until mushrooms release their moisture and begin to brown, about 8-10 minutes.

5. Sprinkle flour over the mushrooms and stir to coat. Cook for 1-2 minutes.

6. Gradually add vegetable broth and almond milk, stirring constantly to prevent lumps.

7. Stir in nutritional yeast and soy sauce. Simmer until the sauce thickens, about 5-7 minutes.

8. Season with salt and pepper to taste.

9. Serve the mushroom stroganoff over cooked pasta.

Serving: Makes 4 servings

Nutrition (per serving, stroganoff only):

Calories: 250

Protein: 8g

Fat: 10g

Carbohydrates: 35g

Fiber: 5g

Sugar: 6g

Sample Meal Plans

12.1 One-week Meal Plan for Beginners

Day 1

- Breakfast: Anti-inflammatory Smoothie
- Lunch: Quinoa Salad with Roasted Vegetables
- Snack: Apple slices with almond butter
- Dinner: Chickpea Spinach Curry with Brown Rice
- Snack: Carrot sticks with hummus

Day 2

- Breakfast: Nutritious Breakfast Bowl
- Lunch: Lentil and Vegetable Soup
- Snack: Mixed nuts and seeds
- Dinner: Baked Salmon with Steamed Broccoli and Quinoa
- Snack: Fresh fruit (apple, orange, or pear)

Day 3

- Breakfast: Avocado Toast on Whole Grain Bread
- Lunch: Chickpea Spinach Salad
- Snack: Greek yogurt with honey and walnuts
- Dinner: Stir-fried Tofu with Vegetables and Brown Rice
- Snack: Celery sticks with almond butter

Day 4

- Breakfast: Chia Seed Pudding
- Lunch: Mediterranean Quinoa Bowl

- Snack: Hummus with bell pepper strips
- Dinner: Vegan Lentil Shepherd's Pie
- Snack: Handful of berries

Day 5

- Breakfast: Smoothie Bowl
- Lunch: Black Bean and Avocado Wrap
- Snack: Edamame
- Dinner: Spaghetti Squash with Tomato Basil Sauce
- Snack: Apple slices with peanut butter

Day 6

- Breakfast: Oatmeal with Fresh Fruit and Nuts
- Lunch: Kale and Quinoa Salad
- Snack: Trail mix (nuts, seeds, dried fruit)
- Dinner: Grilled Chicken with Sweet Potato and Asparagus
- Snack: Sliced bell peppers with guacamole

Day 7

- Breakfast: Greek Yogurt with Berries and Honey
- Lunch: Tomato and Avocado Salad
- Snack: Rice cakes with almond butter
- Dinner: Baked Cod with Quinoa and Steamed Vegetables
- Snack: Fresh fruit salad

12.2 Advanced Meal Plan for Long-term Management

For those who have already adjusted to a diet conducive to managing Giant Cell Arteritis (GCA) and are looking for more advanced meal planning, this guide offers a diverse and nutrient-rich weekly meal plan. This plan is designed to not only provide balanced nutrition but also incorporate a wider variety of anti-inflammatory and nutrient-dense foods to help maintain long-term health and manage GCA effectively.

Day 1

- Breakfast: Green Smoothie with Spirulina
- Lunch: Farro Salad with Roasted Vegetables and Tahini Dressing
- Snack: Beet Hummus with Cucumber Slices
- Dinner: Grilled Lemon Herb Salmon with Quinoa Pilaf
- Snack: Chia Seed Pudding with Berries

Day 2

- Breakfast: Overnight Oats with Almond Butter and Banana
- Lunch: Chickpea and Spinach Stew
- Snack: Roasted Chickpeas
- Dinner: Lentil and Sweet Potato Curry
- Snack: Dark Chocolate and Almonds

Day 3

- Breakfast: Scrambled Tofu with Spinach and Mushrooms
- Lunch: Mediterranean Lentil Salad
- Snack: Apple Slices with Tahini
- Dinner: Stuffed Bell Peppers with Ground Turkey and Brown Rice
- Snack: Mixed Berries

Day 4

- Breakfast: Quinoa Breakfast Bowl with Nuts and Seeds
- Lunch: Butternut Squash Soup with a Side Salad
- Snack: Greek Yogurt with Flaxseeds
- Dinner: Baked Cod with Pesto and Roasted Vegetables
- Snack: Celery Sticks with Hummus

Day 5

- Breakfast: Acai Bowl with Granola and Fresh Fruit
- Lunch: Zucchini Noodles with Avocado Pesto
- Snack: Spiced Pumpkin Seeds
- Dinner: Grilled Chicken with Steamed Broccoli and Cauliflower Rice
- Snack: Pear Slices with Walnuts

Day 6

- Breakfast: Smoothie Bowl with Spinach, Berries, and Chia Seeds
- Lunch: Quinoa and Black Bean Salad with Lime Dressing
- Snack: Edamame
- Dinner: Baked Tofu with Stir-fried Vegetables and Brown Rice
- Snack: Handful of Nuts and Dried Fruit

Day 7

- Breakfast: Chia Pudding with Coconut Milk and Mango
- Lunch: Spinach and Kale Salad with Grilled Chicken and Avocado
- Snack: Carrot Sticks with Almond Butter
- Dinner: Shrimp and Vegetable Skewers with Wild Rice
- Snack: Dark Chocolate Covered Strawberries

This advanced meal plan incorporates a wider variety of anti-inflammatory foods, healthy fats, and lean proteins. The goal is to continue supporting overall health, reduce inflammation, and provide sustained energy levels. Each meal is designed to be nutritionally balanced and flavorful, making long-term dietary adherence more enjoyable and sustainable.

12.3 Exercise For GCA patients

Exercise can help maintain overall health, improve cardiovascular function, and manage the side effects of medications used to treat GCA, such as steroids. Here's a comprehensive exercise routine tailored for GCA patients:

1. Consultation and Personalization

Before starting any exercise routine, GCA patients should consult their healthcare provider. This ensures the exercise plan is safe and tailored to their specific needs, considering the severity of the disease and any other health conditions.

2. Warm-Up (5-10 minutes)

Purpose: To prepare the body for exercise by gradually increasing heart rate and circulation.

- Gentle Walking: Start with a slow walk, gradually increasing the pace.
- Arm Circles: Extend arms out to the sides and make small circles, gradually increasing the size of the circles.
- Neck Stretches: Slowly tilt the head towards each shoulder, hold for a few seconds, and repeat.

3. Cardiovascular Exercise (20-30 minutes)

Purpose: To improve heart and lung function, increase stamina, and aid in weight management.

- Walking: A low-impact exercise that can be done indoors or outdoors. Aim for a brisk pace but avoid overexertion.
- Swimming: Provides a full-body workout with minimal stress on the joints.
- Cycling: Either on a stationary bike or a regular bicycle, at a moderate pace.
- Low-Impact Aerobics: Join a class designed for older adults or beginners.

4. Strength Training (15-20 minutes)

Purpose: To maintain muscle mass, improve joint stability, and enhance overall strength.

- Bodyweight Exercises: Such as squats, lunges, and push-ups. Aim for 2-3 sets of 10-15 repetitions.
- Resistance Bands: Use for exercises like bicep curls, tricep extensions, and shoulder presses.
- Light Weights: Incorporate dumbbells for added resistance. Start with light weights (1-3 pounds) and gradually increase as tolerated.

5. Flexibility and Stretching (10-15 minutes)

Purpose: To maintain joint range of motion, reduce muscle tension, and prevent injury.

- Static Stretching: Hold each stretch for 20-30 seconds. Focus on major muscle groups like hamstrings, quadriceps, calves, and shoulders.
- Yoga: Gentle yoga classes can improve flexibility, balance, and relaxation.
- Tai Chi: A low-impact exercise that combines movement and relaxation, beneficial for balance and flexibility.

6. Balance and Coordination (5-10 minutes)

Purpose: To prevent falls and improve overall stability.

- Standing on One Leg: Hold onto a chair for support if needed. Aim to balance for 10-20 seconds on each leg.
- Heel-to-Toe Walk: Walk in a straight line, placing the heel of one foot directly in front of the toes of the other foot.
- Balance Exercises: Such as side leg raises and toe lifts.

7. Cool Down (5-10 minutes)

Purpose: To gradually lower heart rate and promote relaxation.

- Slow Walking: Gradually decrease the pace of walking.

- Deep Breathing: Inhale deeply through the nose, hold for a few seconds, and exhale slowly through the mouth.
- Gentle Stretching: Repeat some of the stretches from the flexibility section to help relax muscles.

8. Tips for GCA Patients
- Listen to Your Body: Avoid pushing through pain or discomfort. Rest if you feel fatigued or unwell.
- Stay Hydrated: Drink plenty of water before, during, and after exercise.
- Wear Appropriate Footwear: Ensure your shoes provide good support and cushioning.
- Exercise Regularly: Aim for at least 150 minutes of moderate-intensity aerobic activity per week, combined with muscle-strengthening activities on 2 or more days per week.
- Monitor Symptoms: Be aware of any new or worsening symptoms and report them to your healthcare provider.

Regular exercise can significantly benefit GCA patients by enhancing physical and mental health, improving quality of life, and aiding in the management of the condition. Always start slowly, gradually increase intensity, and maintain open communication with your healthcare team to ensure a safe and effective exercise regimen.

Mindful Eating and Lifestyle Tips

13.1 The Importance of Mindful Eating

Mindful eating involves paying full attention to the experience of eating, encouraging a healthier relationship with food. For GCA patients, it can enhance digestion, improve weight management, and reduce stress. By focusing on the sensory aspects of food and recognizing hunger and fullness cues, mindful eating supports better nutritional choices and overall well-being. This practice helps in managing symptoms and side effects of GCA treatments, contributing to a more balanced and enjoyable eating experience.

13.2 Stress Management Techniques

Effective stress management techniques for GCA patients include:

- Mindfulness and Meditation: Practice deep breathing and mindfulness exercises to stay present and calm.
- Physical Activity: Engage in gentle exercises like walking, yoga, or tai chi to reduce stress and improve mood.
- Social Support: Connect with friends, family, or support groups to share experiences and gain emotional support.
- Hobbies and Relaxation: Engage in activities you enjoy, such as reading, gardening, or listening to music, to relax and unwind.

These techniques help manage stress, which can positively impact overall health and well-being.

13.3 Incorporating Physical Activity

Incorporating physical activity for GCA patients can boost overall health and well-being. Start with gentle exercises like walking, swimming, or yoga, gradually increasing intensity as tolerated. Aim for at least 150 minutes of moderate activity per week, and include strength training exercises twice a week. Always consult with a healthcare provider before beginning a new exercise regimen to ensure it aligns with individual health needs. Regular physical activity can improve energy levels, reduce inflammation, and enhance quality of life.